The amazing story of the man who beat cancer three times

Three Battles

by

Russell Currins

Foreword by Ursula Marsden

Published by Russell Currins
Copyright © Russell Currins 2006
All Rights Reserved
This work is Registered with the UK Copyright Service Reg. No. 255813
ISBN: 0-9552550-0-7
From January 1st 2007 ISBN: 978-0-9552550-0-7

All profits from this book will be donated to cancer charities.

Printed by Ripley Printers Ltd

33 Nottingham Road | Ripley | Derbyshire | DE5 3AS

Tel 01773 743621 | Fax 01773 570621

sales@ripleyprinters.com | www.ripleyprinters.com

Acknowledgments

This book is dedicated to a number of people. Firstly, my loving wife Sarah who has stuck by me and given me loving support over the years. My son Dominic who was oblivious to most of it but was a major factor in keeping me going. My family for all their love and support.

I also dedicate this book to many others who have given me support, too many to mention everyone. However of particular mention are the hard working doctors and nurses of the Derbyshire Royal Infirmary and Nottingham City Hospital. Without them I would not have been cured to enable me to write this book.

I also thank my teaching colleagues at Mill Hill School, Ripley, Derbyshire and at Birkdale School, Sheffield who gave great support to us. I am particularly grateful to the support offered by Robert Court, Head Master of Birkdale School and John Turner my teaching colleague in what was also a difficult time for the school during my long absences.

I also thank my colleagues at Birkdale School and our friends at Swanwick Baptist Church for their prayers. We feel they made a difference. I am also grateful to Rev. Roy Plant at the Baptist Church for the visits he made to me in hospital.

There are particular individuals I wish to thank for their help in other ways. Firstly Stephen Gordon, Head of English at Birkdale School for his initial proof reading and editing. I am particularly grateful to Andrea Bevan a professional editor for her advice and suggested changes to ensure this book was produced to a decent standard.

I also express my deepest thanks to Philip and Diane Chadwick and their staff of CDA Creative Communications Ltd. for the book cover design. Sarah and I also thank them for their wonderful support in other ways.

We also thank Nina, our former neighbour and friend who has looked after Dominic on a number of occasions when I was in hospital. Sarah could not have completed her studying without her support.

We are grateful to all our other friends who gave us support or visited me in hospital, particularly John Howell my friend from my school days, Tony Rosser, former colleague at Mill Hill School; Cec Thompson (head of department at my first school) and his wife Anne; Karen; Linda; Alison; friends at Landau; my friend from university Dave and another school friend David.

I also wish to express my gratitude to various retailers who have helped us by providing sales outlets for the book.

Finally I acknowledge the permission given by various people to use their names in this book, particularly doctors who treated me over the years. I give particular thanks to Ursula Marsden and James Hooton from *Emmerdale* for their contribution in terms of the Foreword and permission to use their photograph. In this respect I also thank Stuart Cheetham Researcher for *Emmerdale* for facilitating this.

Back cover picture supplied courtesy of Nottingham Evening Post
Front cover picture courtesy of Derby Evening Telegraph.
Book cover design by CDA Creative Communications Ltd. of Farnsfield,
Nottinghamshire who gave their services free of charge.

FOREWORD

I first came across Russell's book when I was informed by the Emmerdale Research department that some literature had been found on the Internet that might be of some use to me. Feeling an overwhelming sense of responsibility to present viewers with a faithful portrayal of Non Hodgkins Lymphoma through Alice Wilson's storyline I had begun to study its symptoms and the process of CHOP chemotherapy extensively. However, I had only ever experienced the torment of the disease through what my mother in law had reported of her last months with her father in 2000. Thus I knew very little of what it is actually like to live day to day, month to month and often year to year with NHL. Resolved to getting in touch with Leukaemia Research and tentatively asking if one of their team who had survived this rapidly increasing killer would be willing to reveal their family's heartbreak, fears and coping strategies to a complete stranger I decided to put off the call until I had read Three Battles. I recall closing myself in my bedroom (my office) one afternoon last October and emerging hours later in floods of tears at how honest, terrifying and surprisingly amusing in places the Currins family's life with NHL has been. Experiences described such as:

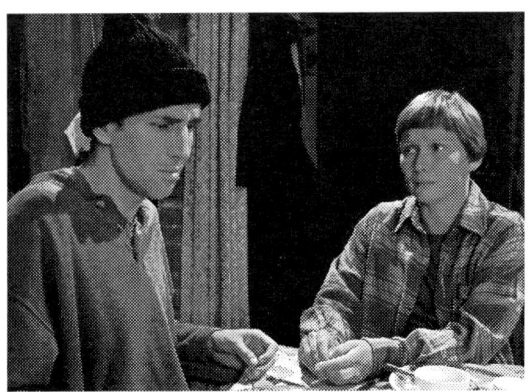

Picture of James Hooton and Ursula Marsden courtesy of ITV Yorkshire

It has also been hurtful to hear stories of people expressing opinions about cancer which were misguided at best, and downright insulting at times. When I chatted to fellow cancer sufferers in clinics and wards I heard many such tales. The most disturbing one was from a lady who was suffering from leukaemia whom I met at Derby. She told me that her neighbour was selling up her house to move away from her because she believed that you could catch cancer like a cold. Words could not describe the anger I felt about this. (Currins:2005)

Became firmly imprinted in my mind and have remained at its forefront throughout my character's journey, not to mention my own. I therefore do not merely recommend Three Battles to you who have, or know someone who has recently been diagnosed with cancer, or to people like myself whose profession has brought him or her into secondary contact with it - I urge you to read this book. Essentially, it will provide insightful factual information that you need to know. Compassionately, it will confirm that sufferers and their families are not alone, that despite there being no cure for Non Hodgkins Lymphoma as yet, there is often light at the end of the tunnel and in the worst possible cases, even if there isn't, life can still be lived and loved to the very, very full.

Ursula Marsden. February 2006

CONTENTS

PREFACE

The book is about my experiences. It is a biography of the events and emotions of being diagnosed with cancer three times and the battle to defeat it again and again. Statistically, about one in three people in the population can expect to be affected by cancer in their lifetime and this often occurs in the later years of life.

However, I am perhaps unique in developing the illness three times but each time I have beaten it and picked up my life again.

I was a schoolteacher for over 20 years, teaching Economics and Business Studies. I spent the first three years of my teaching career at Chesterfield School followed by 13 years as Head of Economics and Business Studies at Mill Hill School, Ripley. My final years were spent as Head of Economics and Business Studies at Birkdale School, Sheffield.

I was first diagnosed in 1995 with Hodgkin's Lymphoma (Lymphocyte Predominant Type) after the discovery of lumps in my neck. I was 35 years old. It was to change my life forever and also the lives of those around me. Thankfully, I was told that it was low-grade and easily curable. After some radiotherapy treatment it was not expected to relapse again and that should have been the end of the story.

However, after five years in remission, in 2001 the disease returned and this time it was more extensive in the bone marrow and the stomach lymph nodes. I received chemotherapy treatment during the autumn of 2001 and the spring of 2002 and was fine for 18 months until a further relapse in October 2003. This time the disease had transformed itself into Non-Hodgkin's Lymphoma and was more high-grade (aggressive). This time I had three courses of intensive chemotherapy including a stem cell transplant.

Eventually, after the third occurrence, I decided to seek retirement as a teacher on medical grounds.

All of this inspired me to write this book which is intended to raise funds for Cancer Research, the Lymphoma Trust Fund at Nottingham City Hospital and the Lymphoma Association. It is also intended to give hope to those who may be diagnosed with such illness in the future that cancer can be beaten. The coming chapters will reveal how that worked for me.

My story will take the reader through the different occurrences of lymphoma. It will discuss the symptoms, the emotional roller-coaster for everyone involved, the treatments, the side-effects and the long-term changes it has made to my life.

Russell Currins
2006

CHAPTER 1
The Seeds of Trouble

My story begins one spring day in 1991. I was shaving and noticed in the mirror a lump in my throat on the right-hand side. It did not look threatening and I thought nothing more about it. Many times after then I regretted not going to my GP at that stage: a visit which might have avoided worse experiences in the future. However I was only 30 years old. Young people don't develop serious illnesses – or so I thought.

I had been a school teacher for eight years. I had been Head of Economics and Business Studies at Mill Hill School, a pleasant, rural school in Ripley, Derbyshire since I was 25 years old. It had been a quick rise to Head of Department. I was originally from Hull but after attending university I settled in Derbyshire when a teaching post became available at Chesterfield School in 1983.

I seemed to be very successful with good examination results and success in extra-curricular activities, particularly a scheme called Young Enterprise. This was a competition where sixth-formers started up and ran their own businesses for one year. They competed with other schools and through my guidance the school had won many trophies over the years. I was hence well regarded by the Head Teacher.

I had married Sarah in 1987. She was from Nottinghamshire and was a hard-working, efficient clerical officer. We shared four happy years of marriage up to 1991. To date there were no children as we both enjoyed our careers and holidays. At the time when I first noticed the lump, life was busy and exciting. I was about to go on holiday to Portugal with Sarah and life was for living. This lump was not bothering me and no-one else seemed to notice it, not even Sarah. Life went on…

That year it was a good summer with excellent weather in the school holidays; a wonderful time for a teacher when you feel that nothing in the world can bother you. I thought nothing more about the lump and it did not seem to change in size or bother me. I also felt very well so there could not be anything wrong.

In November I seemed to notice it again. I had always hated November even though it was the month of my birthday. The nights become very dark with no hope of improvement. I had always been a SAD (Seasonal Affective Disorder) person who found winter difficult and it was a time of year when I worried more about things.

I then started feeling the lump in my neck and although it did not appear to be growing or bothering me in any way it still worried me and I kept feeling it, like a developing habit, hoping it would go away. I also believed, foolishly, that feeling it might somehow make it disappear. One day in the staff room at school one of my colleagues noticed me feeling it and remarked, 'Is your neck swollen?' This filled me with horror! Perhaps it was something more serious because it was noticeable. I did not realise that if you keep feeling a part of your body eventually someone would notice. Feelings of fear and panic came over me with a sinking feeling. I felt that something serious was wrong and that I could do nothing about it.

In response, I started looking at our family medical encyclopaedia. It is often the case that when people are afraid they will try to work out what is the matter themselves, in the hope that, by so doing, they can convince themselves that nothing is wrong. The word 'cancer' came into my head for the first time. I thought, 'surely not'; it did not seem to be growing and it did not hurt. I later discovered that cancerous lumps tend to be painless.

I then had an idea! I could use old photographs to determine whether the lump had suddenly appeared or if it had been there a while. To my relief, looking at old holiday photographs dating back to 1986 it was evident that one side of my neck was swollen compared with the other. The lump was also clearly visible on a photograph taken in Cyprus in 1988. I breathed a sigh of relief! Surely it could not be serious; it had been there a long time. It must be just the way I was. I then went back to the medical encyclopaedia and researched neck problems and it suggested a goitre or thyroid problem or Hodgkin's Disease. I felt sure that it could not be the latter because the lump did not seem to be doing anything or causing any illness. I therefore did not feel it worth visiting my GP and started to lighten up about it. I knew how my body felt. It would be wasting the GP's time.

I had never discussed my fears with Sarah because I knew that she would have sent me off to the doctor immediately whereas I would do anything to avoid the doctor in case he found anything. I also did not want to worry Sarah but during this period I became more bad-tempered which puzzled and upset her. She thought that it was something she had done. However, there was no obvious wrongdoing on her part. When I began worrying about my health I become more withdrawn as a person at home and, because I was not openly discussing it with Sarah, relations between us became strained which almost led to the break-up of our marriage in 1992. However, we stayed together. I eventually became sweeter-tempered and learned an important lesson about being open with Sarah about my worries. Despite this, I still did not tell Sarah of my health fears at that time. I made up an excuse about pressures at work. Teaching was that sort of job so it sounded a viable reason to Sarah for my behaviour. I was to learn a harsher lesson in later years about the importance of not running away from, or dodging, health worries but, rather, meeting them head on.

Life continued and over the next four years I tried to forget about the problem although it remained implanted at the back of my mind. Every day, when I thought that my brain had forgotten about it, it would come back to haunt me.

However, there were major distractions in my life to help me forget. The first was positive. I knew that I needed to move on from my present school if I was to fulfil my potential in the profession. I aimed to become a deputy head or even a head teacher. To achieve this goal I decided to undertake some further study. I firstly attended an information technology course to improve my skills. Many of my pupils knew much more about computers than I did! This set me up for my principal project of gaining a Master of Philosophy degree. This was a higher qualification which I felt was essential if I were to aim at the post of deputy, or head, teacher. I successfully produced a thesis and was awarded the degree by the University of Nottingham in December 1994.

The other distractions in my life were less positive. In November 1992 there was a road-rage incident in which Sarah was injured. I had upset a 'Hell's Angel' biker on the road and, as a result, he stopped his bike in front of my car and smashed the passenger window, resulting in serious cuts to Sarah and a nasty injury to one of her fingers. This caused great psychological upset for a while and lasting damage to Sarah's finger.

Sarah then experienced a period of difficulties at work. She worked in an office environment and there was a feeling of jealously among the other women who worked in her office. She was a glamorous, good-looking woman who liked to present herself well. She had a husband who was a successful teacher which suggested a good standard of living. Sarah felt that she was treated differently from others of her grade by her supervisors because of their jealousy.

Increasingly, Sarah became depressed and by 1993 she wanted to walk away from her work environment and the people who were mentally torturing her. We both went on holiday to Corfu in August to attempt to lift the depression. However, on return to work the feelings of depression were still there and eventually she was presented with a damning, but unfair, appraisal report. One morning in October Sarah experienced hot sweats and could not go into work. She lay on the bed and could scarcely move to do anything. She made an appointment to see her GP and he diagnosed reactive depression and suggested some time off work. In the event, Sarah was off work for four months. Eventually, she showed signs of recovery and sought counselling to help her. This paid off and in February 1994 she returned to work. However, this was in the same office environment as before. The same feelings returned and four weeks later she was presented with another damning appraisal report by her supervisors. This caused great distress once again because it appeared to be unfair.

Sarah was absent from work once more with depression and, in fact, was never to return to the same workplace. She took long-term sick leave with the full support of her GP. However, we both wondered what would be the final outcome.

These events meant that Sarah needed my support. How could I burden her with any health worries I had? They also focused my mind away from my problem for much of the time. By the spring of 1995 Sarah had been on sick leave for over a year. Life was drifting along. Neither of us knew how to resolve Sarah's problem. However, my problem was about to take centre stage.

At the end of the glorious summer of 1995 the lump which I had first noticed in 1991 suddenly appeared to intensify and was about to cause tremendous upheaval in my life. The first battle with cancer was about to begin.

CHAPTER 2
Hodgkin's: the First Time

Almost four years had passed and although periodically I looked at and felt at my neck, I was convinced that nothing was wrong because the lump did not seem to grow. My health also continued to be generally very good. 1995 was an excellent year for me. My school reached the National Final of the Young Enterprise competition. This was a tremendous event with two days in London. It seemed that this might be the break I needed to move my teaching career on. I had been stuck at my present school for too long and I needed to move on to further my ambitions of deputy headship or beyond. Things seemed to be falling into place. After my initial health fears in 1991 I successfully completed a Master of Philosophy research degree between 1992 and 1994, graduating in December 1994 from the University of Nottingham. Little did I know that Nottingham would feature in my life in a different way ten years later.

In 1995 events seemed to be moving in my favour. I had already gained a successful track record as a teacher and the Young Enterprise success might be the final piece of the jigsaw to fulfil my potential. This was followed by a wonderful summer. August 1995 was the hottest on record and life felt good. However my world seemed to be thrown into doubt again when one day I was talking to a neighbour who suddenly remarked that she thought that my neck was swollen. This was the first remark by anyone since 1991. I retorted that my neck had been like this for many years and I did not worry about it. Nothing else was said.

This time I did mention it to Sarah who indicated that she had not noticed any change but I expect if you live with someone (every day) long enough you do not always notice any changes. I thought little more about it and enjoyed the remainder of the summer.

In early September 1995 we paid a visit to my parents in Hull and my mother came out with a remark which shook me. She thought that my neck was swollen and this began a discussion. My mother was and still is very intuitive with regard to the welfare of myself and my two brothers. She often said that a mother's love is special and it enables her to tune in to anything wrong with her children.

Sarah promised my mother that I would be visiting our GP as soon as we returned home. I then looked at my neck again and for the first time became convinced myself that the lump had grown and the side of my neck appeared to be swollen. I went back to the medical encyclopaedia and was drawn to Hodgkin's Disease, a cancer of the lymphatic system. The book also indicated that it was highly curable if treated early. I then regretted not having it dealt with in 1991. I hoped that it was not too late.

As promised I visited my GP, Dr Skidmore, about the middle of September. He looked at the lump and the swollen side of the neck, measured it and wrote down some details. He displayed no expression and gave no indication as to what it might be. Dr Skidmore is a wonderful GP; he has been extremely good to my wife through her illness (which is discussed in the next chapter). He did exactly the best thing and stated that he would send me to a specialist and asked if the Derbyshire Royal Infirmary was acceptable. We lived in the middle of Derbyshire with a choice of four hospitals. I knew little about any of them and took his advice. My long association with the Derbyshire Royal Infirmary (DRI) was about to begin.

Upon returning home I informed Sarah of all of this. She comforted me but I could tell there was a worried look on her face. However, she thought that because the swollen neck had been there so long it must be a cyst or something. I felt very low in spirit and deep down I suspected it was cancer. I felt that I was never going to be the same person ever again and all my hopes for the future were in ruins. However, I consoled myself with fact that I felt well and therefore surely it could not be too serious. There are other symptoms associated with lymphoma cancers such as night sweats, fever, loss of appetite, weight loss, tiredness, a cough and breathlessness. I had none of these and actually felt very well.

On 3 October, 1995 I visited the DRI for the first time to see Mr Parker, Consultant for Ear, Nose and Throat problems. Dr Skidmore suggested that I take the photographs showing the lump in previous years. Mr Parker appeared to be a very knowledgeable doctor in his field and there were three student doctors in the room. They all had a feel of the lump, which in fact turned out to be three, in the throat! Mr Parker gave some words of assurance after looking at the photographs that because it had been there for so long it was unlikely to be life threatening. He did state, however, that there would be a MRI (Magnetic Resonance Imaging) scan and a biopsy on one of the lumps to assess exactly what was going on. This took place about two weeks after the initial appointment with Mr Parker. It involved producing magnetic images of the neck and head rather than conventional X-rays. The MRI scan is an unpleasant experience where your head is enclosed in a closed tunnel. Although it is a relatively safe scan, involving magnetic imaging rather than X-rays, nevertheless, it is an experience which would be difficult for anyone who does not like to feel enclosed.

In the meantime, while waiting for scans, I tried to get on with my life, having great faith in Mr Parker's ability to sort the problem out. I still had career ambitions and at this stage could see no reason why I should not continue to look for jobs. You cannot put your life on hold for something which might never happen.

A great opportunity had come up in the September for a post as Regional Development Advisor with BTEC for Business. This would be based in Nottingham and would involve travelling around schools in the East Midlands helping to set up and inspect GNVQ courses at schools and colleges. This was the kind of higher status post which I had longed for and now, just when it seemed within my grasp, it appeared that I was to be denied.

I applied for the post and was successful in gaining a first interview in London. This happened after I had seen Mr Parker for the first time. It was a very pleasant experience. Sarah came down to London with me and afterwards we had a wonderful meal in a friendly Italian restaurant in Farringdon. I was confident of a second interview and this duly followed on 30 October. This was to be a two-day event with an overnight stay at the Charing Cross Hotel in the executive suite. Sarah was allowed to come along so we made it into a short break since it was half-term. However, by the time the second interview finally arrived events had taken a more uncertain turn with my health.

In between the interviews I had been to a second clinic appointment, seeing a very pleasant Registrar on 24th October. He had the results of the MRI scan. It showed many

16

more lumps than I had expected. There was a large lump in my throat but also many lumps around the side of my neck, which looked like a bag of peas. The Registrar stated that they now proposed to conduct a biopsy on the large lump in the throat. It was to take place through an aspiration test. This involved inserting a needle into the lump to draw out cells which could then be examined. It was hoped that this would avoid the need for surgery. This was to take place on 3 November.

I therefore now faced the second interview for the BTEC post not knowing what the future would hold. I was placed in a terrible dilemma. If I was successful in gaining the post in Nottingham I would have to resign from my school on 31 October because the post was due to start in January 1996. However, what if I had developed a serious illness and consequently needed sick leave in my new post? I would probably be dismissed for not informing BTEC and would have no job. I did not know what to do. My first thought was to withdraw from the interview but Sarah suggested that I speak to my Headmaster. He was very sympathetic and helped resolve the dilemma by allowing me an extension of the resignation deadline to the middle of November. By then I would have the results of the aspiration test and could withdraw from the BTEC post and still have a job at Mill Hill School if the illness turned out to be serious.

I therefore went down to London on 30 October but although I enjoyed the experience I did not really perform as well as I could have done because of the worries about my health. Hence, I was not offered the post which was a relief in one way. However, at this point in time I felt very depressed. I felt that the last opportunity to fulfil my potential had gone. As a result I would now be stuck in teaching and would probably not progress any higher. I felt very hard done by. Why had I been dealt such a bad set of cards? However, later on I would meet other patients who were worse off than me and this feeling would fade.

November 3rd came and I went for the aspiration test at the DRI. Dr Robinson, a specialist Histopathologist, produced a huge needle and stated quite confidently that it would not require a local anaethestic. I wished that I could believe him! I did not realise that our paths would cross again eight years later when I suffered a relapse. I waited with trepedation for the needle. It hurt for a few seconds but it was not too bad. I was then asked to ring the Ear, Nose and Throat department later on for some results. In fact, I received a telephone call from the Registrar. He informed me that the cells did not reveal anything active but all the cells looked the same which concerned them. He then proposed removing one of the lumps for a biopsy - this would involve a four day stay in hospital.

The thought of a hospital stay numbed me. I had never been in hospital before in my life. I also started to think about the disruption it would cause everyone. I was told that I would need to take two weeks off work. As Head of Economics and Business this thought horrified me because so many people depended on me. At least I had time to prepare as I was given a date of 20 November for the biopsy.

As the weekend before the biopsy approached I was filled with apprehension. It was ironic that I had never felt fitter in my life. I even chopped branches off a tree in the garden, thinking that it would be the last opportunity for a while. I asked myself why I was going into hospital when I felt so well. This is the irony about cancer. The patient can feel very well in the early stages and not even realise they have the disease.

Eventually Monday 20 November came. Sarah took me down to the DRI for 8.00 a.m. We reported in and were taken up to Ward 32 at the top of the building, with excellent views of Derby. Then came the waiting game, which is the worst experience of any operation. At 9.00 the Registrar came to see me and suggested that they would take a small lump at the back of the neck for a biopsy. He warned that this could cause a problem with a tendon and make stretching difficult. This thought did not please me but I trusted that the doctors knew what they were doing.

About 9.30 a.m. the anaesthetist came to see me and explained the procedure. There was then a consent form to sign and I was then asked if I wanted a 'pre-med' to settle me. This is a sedative to calm a patient before an operation. I felt pretty calm but decided it was perhaps a good idea.

Eventually, after what seemed a long time, the theatre staff came to collect me. I remember being wheeled along long corridors and finally delivered to a room with other similar trolleys. I was quite calm but I wondered what was going through Sarah's mind. Later on she described the feelings of sadness and uncertainty as she drove away from the hospital. On the car radio it was playing 'Hard to Say I'm Sorry' by Chicago. One of the lines says, 'After all that we've been through I will make it up to you'. Although Sarah had done nothing to be sorry about, it seemed an appropriate song to express her feelings at that moment.

When I reached the operating theatre I was then given a cap to put on for theatre before being wheeled into a room where the anaesthetist was waiting with his assistants. He then attempted to insert the cannula into a vein in my hand. This is a needle and tube where blood can be taken and drugs can be administered as needed. He remarked about my lack of veins. It was not to be the last time my veins were to cause problems for a nurse or doctor! Eventually, after the cannula was successfully inserted, I was told that I would go to sleep and know nothing. True enough, I went into a deep sleep.

When I woke up I had an oxygen mask over my face and was told by theatre nurses that I had done very well. I was then approached by Mr Parker, the Consultant who had performed the surgery. He informed me that he had removed the large lump at the front and two smaller ones attached to it. At this point I also discovered that there was a tube sticking out of my neck with a bottle to collect any blood from the wound.

I was then taken back to the ward in a daze and put back on my bed to recover. I then slept for another hour or so. When I awoke again I realised that I'd had nothing to eat or drink that morning (nil by mouth). I asked for water and was also brought a cup of tea. Sarah then appeared with some fruit and my favourite rum truffle chocolates. I ate one straight away; it was heaven! I then began to come to life and felt so happy that the operation was all over. At this point I did not worry about what the biopsy results would bring.

When Sarah came to see me she admitted that she was unprepared for the sight of the tube and bottle. Sarah thought that I looked like something out of a *Hammer House of Horror* movie!

Later that day I was moved to a side room, probably to reduce the risk of infection in the wound in the neck. This was wonderful. I had my own TV and pictures on the wall! I can remember this day well because that evening there was the now-famous interview between Princess Diana and Martin Bashir, with the revelations of adultery and the royal marriage problems.

I spent a further three days on Ward 32 in my little room being well looked after. I thought little about the biopsy outcome but Sarah did ask the House Officer who told her that the large lump which had been removed did look suspicious. This upset her afterwards. She confessed later that she had cried a few tears that night but she never showed anything in front of me. Driving home from the hospital that night was a total blur. She was completely shaken. At that point she did not realise that cancers can be cured and that they do not signal an automatic death sentence.

When I came home I picked up very quickly and received an appointment to attend the Ear, Nose and Throat clinic for the biopsy results. To my horror, the appointment was for 29 November, my 35th birthday. How could they do this to me?

We turned up dutifully on the day. Before we went in I could see Mr Parker with his nurse, who was to take the stitches out of my neck during the appointment. They looked our way with very serious faces so I guessed the worst.

We were eventually called in after what seemed an eternity. The nurse began to remove the stitches. At the same time Mr Parker explained that the lump had shown signs of low-level Hodgkin's Disease, a cancer of the lymph glands.

I was not really surprised but it is still numbing to receive such news. That morning I had prayed that it would not be that outcome, but this time my prayer was not answered. However, he softened the blow by stating that if one is going to get a cancer then this is the one to have because it is very curable.

The nurse noticed that it was my birthday and wished me a happy birthday. Mr Parker added that I should expect to celebrate many more. It was not a cancer that would eat away at me. He then stated that I was to be passed on to the Oncology department who would deal with my treatment.

Despite these comforting words it was not the happiest of birthdays. It was made worse when my parents telephoned me that evening as they always did on my birthday. When I mentioned the word cancer to my mother she took it badly and assumed that I was going to die. Many people think that having cancer is always a death sentence but it is not. Thankfully my grandma was there to provide a rock for my mother. She had lost her eldest son, aged 29 years, in 1970. She told my mother to be strong and said, 'I lost my son, you are not going to lose yours!' Sadly, my grandma was no longer with us when I relapsed in later years.

Just to complete the birthday Sarah ordered an Indian take-away for that evening. Even that became lost en route!

It was not easy news to take but at least we were comforted by the fact that it was low-level, and curable. In the following week we met Dr Gillian Thomas, Consultant Oncologist, for the first time. She was very pleasant and upbeat. I was told that I would be having further blood tests, a bone marrow biopsy and a CT scan to assess whether or not it had spread elsewhere. She expected the results to be negative but they had to be sure.

I was then sent for blood tests the same day and was given appointments for the bone marrow biopsy and CT scan. The biopsy was conducted by Dr Grant who was to be in charge of my treatment when I relapsed with the disease the next time. I knew nothing of what the biopsy would entail which was just as well! Dr Grant produced a variety of ominous-looking surgical instruments and asked me to lie on my side on the bed.

She gave me a local anaesthetic which was painful in itself and then proceeded to do what felt like drilling into my pelvic bone. The pain was excruciating but Sarah held my hand. I remember this painful experience well. Since then, when requiring a biopsy, I have always taken the offer of a sedative. I am a coward when it comes to pain!

After the biopsy was over Dr Grant showed me the sample. It looked like a thin piece of meat in a clear fluid. Two days later came the CT scan (sometimes called a CAT scan). This is a sophisticated type of X-ray which builds up a three-dimensional picture of the inside of the body and can detect abnormal growths.

Before I arrived I was asked not to eat or drink anything for four hours. Upon arrival I was asked to drink a grey-looking drink which tasted like aniseed; this was to help the results from the scan show up. After four cups I was asked to change into an operating gown and then led into a room with a large-looking machine with an arch. Thankfully, I was not to be enclosed as with the MRI scan. I was asked to lie flat on a long table and given an injection of a dye, again to help show up the results. The dye had strange side-effects, such as making the patient feel hot flushes and a desire to go to the toilet.

The table moved up and down and I heard the whirr of the machine. At regular intervals I was asked to breathe in and hold my breath. Thankfully, someone remembered to tell me to breathe normally as well! Afterwards I was told that I might need the toilet. This was the understatement of the day!

With all biopsies and scans completed we had another appointment with Dr Thomas on 18 December, 1995. She was smiling and informed us that the bone marrow, CT scans and blood tests were all fine. I had Hodgkin's Disease in the lymph nodes of the neck only. It was a low-grade, slow-growing type 1A called Lymphocyte Predominant which is actually rare (about 5% of cases) but easily curable. There are four stages of development of lymphoma cancers and, thankfully, mine was only at the first stage this time and confined to one area of the body. However, in the later relapses it was to become more extensive.

This was excellent news after weeks of uncertainty. I was to be given a course of radiotherapy over four weeks to shrink the remaining lumps in the neck. This was such a relief to Sarah and I because we had wanted to start a family in 1995. We had married in 1987 but had never really been enthusiastic about having any children before this time. We both had our careers and enjoyed our holidays and freedom. We expressed our relief to Dr Thomas about the fact that I was not going to receive chemotherapy because we both knew the implications this could have for conceiving babies. Both of our spirits lifted. Dr Thomas smiled and said the treatment should have no effect on my fertility and grinned as she told me, 'Get conceiving'.

This was not something we could do initially because all the stress of the preceding few weeks had inflamed Sarah's endometriosis. This is a condition in women which can result in infertility. Sarah had first been treated for this condition in 1994 but it seemed to return during the stressful period of my operation, scans and treatment. She was now given another course of treatment and, later in the year, we were successful in conceiving our first child. Before that happened, however, there was the radiotherapy treatment to undergo.

CHAPTER 3

Treatment the First Time

In January 1996 I began my first course of radiotherapy. I had heard of other people having such treatment and wondered with trepidation what was in store.

Before treatment could begin there was a preparation process which proved surprisingly involved. This began at the end of December 1995. The radiotherapy would be concentrated on the areas where the tumours were and lymph glands under my right arm to prevent a spread of any cancerous cells. I was informed that I would need to wear a specially-made mask to protect all other areas of my chest and head. Radiotherapy is a treatment where powerful X-rays are focused on the cancerous cells with the aim of destroying them. However, without protection other areas of the body can be damaged. The mask proved to be a surprisingly unpleasant experience. The radiographer who was producing the mask put what seemed like a cloth over my face and chest followed by a moist, clay-like material which moulded itself to the contours of my body. This was disconcerting because my eyes were covered so I was in darkness.

The radiographer then proceeded to provide a lecture about how cancers are caused by people abusing their bodies, e.g., too much sunlight or smoking. However, this was not what I wanted to hear and when I challenged him he could not explain what caused Hodgkin's Disease!

It seems ironic that I had never really abused my body. I have never smoked. I was never a big drinker, even in my student days. My only vice was enjoying the sun and holidays in hot places. I always believed that I would be a candidate for skin cancer if anything, and if that happened then it would be my own fault; I thought there was no reason why I should have developed Hodgkin's Disease and it did not seem fair. However, this form of cancer can happen to anyone. I was later told that it was not due to anything that I had done or not done. It was just one of those things that happen to some people in life. Sarah and I both believe that events in life happen for a reason but at that moment I could not think why I should have developed Hodgkin's Disease.

Once the mask was made there were further hospital appointments to fit it and to set the X-ray co-ordinates. These took place over a two-week period at the beginning of January 1996.

Treatment was initially scheduled for 17 January (ironically, my brother's birthday and also the anniversary of when I had an impacted wisdom tooth removed in 1991). However, I asked for a week's delay; this was because one of my students had been invited to London to receive the BTEC Student of the Year Runner-Up prize for Business. This was to be awarded by the Duke of Kent and, as the student's teacher, I was invited as well. This was too good an opportunity to miss. It is not every day that you get to meet the Duke of Kent. Despite my illness, I seemed to have a habit of meeting famous people over the years. I once sat next to Bruce Grobbelar, the famous goalkeeper at a restaurant in Liverpool in 1992. I had earlier met Michael Heseltine at the Young Enterprise National Final in 1995. In later years, I was to meet Eric Clapton. It is strange how life can swing from highs to lows in short spaces of time.

Dr Thomas was prepared to agree to this delay because mine was a low-level lymphoma. One week would not really make any difference, so my radiotherapy treatment finally began on 22 January, 1996. I was given a slot to attend for Monday to Friday for four weeks. Each time I arrived I was asked to lie on a table; the mask was fitted and then I heard the whirring of the machine which rotates around you. When the X-rays were administered the sound was like that of a microwave oven, and the process took about three minutes. Afterwards, the mask was removed and I went home until my slot the next day.

The same routine continued over the next four weeks, except for the odd occasion when treatment was postponed when the machine broke down. Eventually, on 21 February, the final treatment was completed.

I had been counting down the days with the help of a bag of £1 coins. Car parking was £1 per day so as the coins went down I knew that my treatment was coming to an end. At the finish I brought in a card and a box of chocolates as a thank you to the team of radiographers who had been dealing with my treatment. I was then given an appointment to see Dr Thomas the following week.

During the treatment I could feel the remaining lumps in my neck disappearing. At the finish my neck was normal and Dr Thomas's first remark was, 'How do you like your new neck?' I felt elated that it was over and especially so since she indicated that there was only a 1-3% chance of the disease returning.

I felt that I had been very lucky in this respect. It could have been much worse. However, there was a sting in the tail. A week after completing treatment my neck had a 'sunburn' line down the middle. This was very sore and felt exactly as if I had been badly sunburnt. It was highly visible after the February half-term and colleagues at school had looks of horror on their faces. Thankfully, the soreness died down after a week and I was then left with a golden suntan down one side of my neck. I was also left with a more horrible legacy.

Radiotherapy is a blunt instrument and it left me with an area of my neck without hair. It looked as though a wedge had been taken out by a clumsy hairdresser. I now had a designer haircut which was never really to grow back properly. This was something I had to live with. My hairline was now shorter on one side of my neck than the other. What would people think? In the event no-one ever said anything but I was always conscious of the 'wedge' which has never grown back properly to this day. In later years I was to develop red blotches on my neck and at the top of the shoulder next to the neck. This was long-term skin damage from the radiotherapy although I do not blame anyone, it was a necessary evil.

Later on, I was placed on three-monthly checks with Dr Thomas. From 1996 to 2001 the disease did not recur. Blood tests were always consistent and the lumps never returned. Sarah and I were able to get on with our lives. Dr Thomas had already indicated that there was only a small chance of it returning and reassured me that if it did they would cure it again. Sarah told me that she never gave it another thought and always believed it would never come back. Once again, I felt very lucky compared with others who I had met.

Life now moved on. We booked a late holiday to Menorca in April and then had friends stay with us from the Crimea. In August of 1996 we were fortunate enough for Sarah to become pregnant and after a reasonably straightforward pregnancy our son, Dominic, was born on 16 April 1997. At this point we really believed that Hodgkin's Disease was behind us and we could look forward to a happier period in our lives with our son and, hopefully, more children.

Unfortunately life is rarely like that. Two weeks after Dominic was born Sarah became ill and it took about two and half years for her to pick up. She was eventually diagnosed with Chronic Fatigue Syndrome and she had developed a wheat or gluten allergy. These were difficult times when I had to do more for Dominic than the average father. During this period I rarely thought about my own disease; I had my regular check ups which were always fine.

Eventually, by the autumn of 1999, Sarah's health picked up and on 5 December 1999 we finally had Dominic christened. Also, as Sarah's health improved, I felt confident enough to look at resurrecting my teaching career. I applied for two jobs and was invited to interviews. The first job was a Head of Faculty at a school in Nottinghamshire but it wasn't really what I wanted. However on 7 July I was invited for interview at Birkdale School, an independent school in Sheffield. To my surprise, I was offered the post on 13 July. I regarded this as a step up for me; my new position was to begin on 1 January 2000. Although Sarah was pleased for me, she told me afterwards that it planted seeds of doubt in her mind about whether the commuting to and from Sheffield would prove too much and damage my health.

However, Sarah and I both began the new century and millennium with great hope for the future. Dominic began nursery school and showed signs of being a bright boy. In fact, 2000 was a good year. The job began well at Birkdale and I felt that it had been a good move. On 29 November I celebrated my 40th birthday. Truly, I thought, life begins at 40 and I felt that we could expect many happy years ahead.

CHAPTER 4
Life Begins at Forty

It was a very good first year at Birkdale School. Exam results were good and the school gained Young Enterprise success, winning the Sheffield Area Best Company award in my first year. There was also an inspection during the first weeks of my time at Birkdale and this seemed to go really well. I had reached my 40th birthday and felt reasonably content with life. Birkdale was an excellent school to work in. It had a deep Christian ethos and set high expectations for its pupils. Most pupils had an excellent attitude and gained first class examination results.

However, there were signs of problems developing. The Upper and Lower Sixth Business sets had a sprinkling of students who seemed to be less motivated than others in the school. This was unusual for Birkdale, I was surprised to discover that not all students in an independent school automatically work hard and yet some parents expect results nonetheless.

At the beginning of 2001 Sarah, Dominic and I started the year with a relaxing holiday in Lanzarote. It was the first time we had taken a winter holiday and it was wonderful. However, Sarah noticed that I did not have as much energy as usual. I had also developed a cough after a strange cold in the previous December which would not go away even after we had escaped the British winter for a week. Sarah made me go to see our GP towards the end of January.

Dr Skidmore prescribed some penicillin for what appeared to be a chest infection. It seemed to ease a little but did not clear completely and in March I went back and was prescribed some stronger antibiotics. Despite these, the cough never really fully cleared up but I did not want to keep going back for more antibiotics. I did not think there was anything significant about it and believed it would clear up in the Spring.

All of this coincided with an unhappy term at Birkdale when I felt under some pressure. In January 2001 there was an unexpectedly low set of grades for A level Business Studies coursework. This had been marked externally and I was perplexed as to why they were so low. I attempted to gain feedback from the Board as to why but little was forthcoming which caused stress. I felt under pressure to obtain more information because of a number of grumbles from parents.

To further add to the stress there were incidents of immature behaviour and lack of effort from elements of both Business Studies groups. I did not discuss this with my line manager because I had not been in the job very long and did not want to give the impression that I could not deal with such pupils. The school was very supportive to its staff but it was my pride that prevented me seeking help. However I did request that the Upper Sixth group be split to provide better support but this was not possible because of timetabling constraints. The group was too large in my opinion and did not have a good attitude to work.

These events seemed to start grinding me down, and for the first time in my teaching career I felt my confidence draining. Not much seemed to be going right and I could not seem to motivate pupils as well as I had done at my previous school.

I felt so stressed that we booked another holiday, in Gran Canaria, for the Easter holiday in April 2001. The cough persisted on holiday even though the weather was hot. Sarah also noticed that I could not seem to take the heat as I usually did; I normally thrived in hot climates.

After returning to school there was a great deal of work because my colleague and I were pushing the Upper Sixth for their A levels but also preparing the Lower Sixth for the first AS level examinations. I also had another check up for Hodgkin's Disease in April. When I attended there was a surprise. Dr Thomas had suddenly moved on. The locum doctor indicated that all was well; blood tests were normal and there were no lumps. Dr Thomas had recommended before she left that I be placed on annual check-ups from this point onwards which was excellent news. I mentioned the cough. The locum doctor ordered a chest X-ray but this was clear so he was happy with my health.

However I felt that Dr Thomas moving on was a bad omen. I did not really feel fully well but at this stage never contemplated that it might be the return of Hodgkin's disease in a different form.

My health seemed to improve during the year and I felt much better in May and early June. I assumed that this was because my tiresome Upper Sixth Business Studies group had left and things were easier because the Lower Sixth were on study leave for AS examinations. However towards the end of June I started to feel fatigued and developed a thirst which I could never seem to quench. It was very noticeable on 30 June when Sarah, Dominic and I went to Sheffield to the Birkdale School summer fair. We had lunch on the way home. I had two large orange juices to drink and still felt very thirsty. Sarah also noticed that my appetite was less than usual. It was a fine day but not hot so these symptoms were unlikely to be due to the weather.

As July progressed the symptoms continued and were compounded by an additional problem which developed, of impotence, which started to put some pressure on my relationship with Sarah. I could not understand what was wrong and, unfortunately, the only explanation I could offer Sarah was that it had been a stressful year. However, she did not really accept this since there had been periods of stress before in my teaching career which had not appeared to cause such a problem. We later discovered that it was the cancer returning which was the cause.

When the summer holiday arrived these symptoms continued. On one occasion when my brother and his girlfriend came to stay I felt so tired I just lay on the floor. I did not need telling to go to see my GP, particularly in view of the impotence problem. Dr Skidmore thought that I was badly stressed and that things would improve, including the cough which was still there a little. He told me to come back if things did not improve. They did not, so the following week I went back to the surgery but Dr Skidmore was on holiday, so I saw a locum. Of course, he knew little of my medical history and he seemed concerned when questioning me about my health when I revealed the history of Hodgkin's Disease.

He then ordered a whole range of blood tests to test the various body functions including blood counts, glucose levels, liver function and kidney function. At this stage, I thought that I was becoming diabetic because of the thirst and tiredness. Sarah thought it was a virus and was even afraid that I had developed Chronic Fatigue Syndrome, the symptoms of which she was familiar with. At this time I was drinking about three glasses of water at the end of the day and would go to the toilet more often. Sarah was very worried but at this stage the word 'cancer' did not appear in her head. I, too, did not have the slightest suspicion that it was the return of Hodgkin's Disease.

When I telephoned the surgery to check if the test results had come back I was told to make an appointment to see Dr Skidmore because he needed to discuss the results with me. When he gave me the results it emerged that my red blood count was low so I was anaemic. I was also informed that my kidneys were failing. This was because the level of calcium salts in my kidneys was too high. I did not even know what he meant by calcium salts, although I deduced that high levels of salts might explain the thirst.

Dr Skidmore remarked that I was anaemic, just as was the Queen Mother, an item in the news at the time. He had also looked back at the blood counts (which had been sent to him) from previous check-ups at the Derbyshire Royal Infirmary and noticed that my red blood count had been falling steadily from 1997 to 2001 which puzzled him, although it had always remained within normal range until now. He considered what to do and indicated that I would be referred back to Oncology at Derby and I received an appointment for the following week.

At this stage I still did not contemplate a return of Hodgkin's Disease because I could feel no lumps on the outside of my body. This view was shared by Dr Grant, the Consultant I went to see on 7 August 2001. Although in no way her fault, I had unhappy memories of Dr Grant because she had conducted the first, painful, bone marrow biopsy in 1995.

I was dubious about having an appointment on the 7th day of the month; for some reason, the number 7 had not always been lucky for me even though I had been for interview at Birkdale School on 7 July and at the time considered that to have been a positive day. However, judging from the difficult year I was having at Birkdale I was beginning to doubt that it had been the right move and perhaps 7 July 1999 had not been so lucky after all. Another less than happy association was 7 November 1992 when Sarah had been attacked by a 'Hells Angel' in a road rage incident.

However, I still did not expect cancer and, after examining me, Dr Grant stated that 'If it was lymphoma it did not jump out at you', because there were no visible lumps in any lymph glands, as in 1995. Also that day Sarah and I met Alan Bryan for the first time. He was a specialist cancer charge nurse and was to feature a great deal in my treatments over the next few years.

Dr Grant was puzzled and sent me the same day for some more blood tests at Derby and then we went home. Nothing could have prepared Sarah and I for the drama of the next day.

On 8 August at about 11.30 a.m. I received a telephone call from Alan Bryan from the DRI. He stated that the blood test results had revealed that the calcium salts in my kidneys were dangerously high. I needed to be admitted to hospital straight away because there was a danger of renal (kidney) failure.

Sarah and I were stunned because we did not realise what it would mean. I packed a bag. Sarah was perhaps in a worse state of shock than me so I agreed to drive her car down to the hospital. On top of everything else, on the way a lorry shunted into the back of Sarah's car at a roundabout in Derby. Thankfully, it was not serious and no-one was hurt but it certainly added to the tension of the day.

On arrival at the Derbyshire Royal Infirmary I was admitted to Ward 10 which was a Haematology ward rather than Oncology. It was a place I was to become very familiar with. However, it was not my first visit. In 1996, after I was in remission the first time, after a clinic visit Sarah and I visited a former colleague from Mill Hill School. He had just been admitted with leukaemia and it was very serious. He later died in 1998 after a relapse. I never believed back then that I would be admitted to the same ward in later years.

I was allocated a side room which was a pleasant surprise but I still had no idea what to expect. Sarah and I were introduced to a friendly registrar called Dr Moorby and a young houseman who we all named Dr Bill. Dr Bill inserted a cannula into my hand to take blood and for drips which were to become become a way of life. Blood was taken and then a drip of saline was set up to get fluids into me because I was actually dehydrating. When you have renal failure (strangely enough) your body cannot hold fluids and you pay more visits to the toilet.

Then Dr Moorby came to see me and he told me that he suspected that the Hodgkin's Disease had returned. This was a huge shock both to Sarah and to me. How could this be? I had only just been put onto annual check-ups that April! Dr Moorby stated that he would perform a bone marrow biopsy because it was suspected that the cancer was now in the bone marrow and this was producing the excess of calcium salts. Sarah was devastated. It had never occurred to her for one minute that the illness would come back. She was also worried about how on earth she would cope with a four-year-old and not being a well person herself, and with no family support. Sarah felt so alone. Luckily her best friend Karen was very supportive as she had been in 1997/98 when Sarah had been very ill.

The bone marrow biopsy was carried out on the afternoon of 8 August. I was offered a sedative which I accepted gratefully, remembering the pain of the previous occasion of such a biopsy. The sedative meant that I remembered nothing about what took place but then Dr Moorby informed Sarah that the bone marrow sample did not come away easily which was not a good sign. Two days later I had a CT scan to assess if there were any signs of cancer elsewhere. In the night, I lay in the hospital bed thinking of poor Sarah at home alone and what she must be going through on her own with a lively four-year-old. Her own health was not perfect even though she had come a long way since Dominic was born. I was her rock and I wondered how she would cope. In addition, Sarah had the extra burden of sorting out the insurance and repair of her car after the accident.

In fact, we were both experiencing a great deal of shock and uncertainty and emotions were running high. When Sarah came to see me on 9 August she was further shocked to find me in the middle of a blood transfusion. I was told that my red blood count had fallen to 8.9 making me very anaemic. (The normal range is 11.5-15.) This set off all sorts of fears and we were frightened that perhaps it was leukaemia, knowing that this results in red blood counts falling very low.

Sarah was not expecting this. We also had a lively four-year-old running around; I had to prevent Dominic pulling the tubes in my hand! Sarah was very emotional. Sometimes she would go out of the room to get a drink and gather her composure because she did not want me to see her upset. She was helped that afternoon by a visit from Catherine who worked for the Chaplaincy service. She came in to see us and, having had health problems herself in the past, was able to empathise with our situation and offer some comfort. Sarah and I were afraid of the unknown and we needed someone like Catherine.

We did have some relief later that afternoon when Dr Moorby told us that they suspected Hodgkin's' Disease which could be cured, but it was not proven at this stage. It certainly was not leukaemia.

By Friday 10 August my kidneys were improving with the saline drips and the steroids I was given. The level of calcium salts was falling and I was able to go home after the CT scan. I was instructed to drink a lot and come back a week later for the results of the biopsies and scan.

I returned to hospital on Thursday 16 August and reported to the Day Case Unit of Ward 10. We met a specialist nurse called Kate who told us that Hodgkin's Disease had been confirmed but she was very positive. She said it was easily treatable.

This was what we needed to hear. Dealing with cancer is all about being positive and you need positive people around you. Kate was joined by Dr Moorby who confirmed what Kate had said and stated that this time it would require chemotherapy treatment. However, he stressed that it was not a nasty chemotherapy and although there would be some hair loss it would not be total. I was also told that my calcium salt level was rising again so I was given some more steroids to take home for the weekend. I was also to come to clinic on the following Tuesday and the intention was to start the chemotherapy the following week.

Knowing that I would need chemotherapy made Sarah feel upset. It was not only because I would suffer side-effects but also, we had wanted another child. Unfortunately I was unable to produce a sperm sample to store. Since my fertility would be reduced we both realised it was unlikely that we would now have any more children. Sarah felt cheated after all that we had been through. It did not seem fair as she had started to feel a little better and felt able to have another pregnancy.

When Sarah and I came to clinic on Tuesday 21 August we were seen by Alan and Dr Grant. We expected confirmation of everything we had been told. However, there was a new shock; we were told that the CT scan had revealed swollen internal stomach lymph nodes as well as the disease being in the bone marrow. There was clearly work to be done. I just wanted to get on with it.

CHAPTER 5
Let Battle Commence

I desperately wanted to fight this illness and begin the chemotherapy as soon as possible. However, before this happened I had another unexpected one-night stay in hospital on 23 August. Blood tests on the 21st had revealed a high level of calcium salts again which needed to be brought down before treatment could begin; it was vital that the kidneys should be functioning fully to discharge the waste from the chemotherapy. Again I was put on saline drips and given a steroid. This time I was given a bed in an open bay of Ward 10 which resulted in a less pleasant stay. Ward 10, being mainly a Haematology ward, dealt with blood disorders but it also dealt with strokes and respiratory problems. As a result it could be noisier, with people coughing and the odd confused or elderly patient on the move in the night trying to shift your belongings off your table! Sometimes it could be amusing, such as when a confused, elderly patient believed the television in the bay was his and why were other patients watching it? He then proceeded to attempt to pick it up to take it away before nurses rushed in to stop him.

Whilst aware that these poor souls could not help themselves it nevertheless made me hope even more that my stay would be a short one.

The doctors planned to begin the chemotherapy on 24 August. However, they still were not happy with my kidney function and sent me to ultrasound to check for any blockages in my tubes. It was important that the tumours in my stomach were not pressing on my urinal tubes preventing the flow of urine because the kidneys needed to be able to dispose of any waste from the chemotherapy. This gave me the opportunity to view them as they showed up as black blobs on the screen. The ultrasound doctor then gave me the green light for the chemotherapy as urine was clearly able to flow. Unfortunately, there was then a delay while the chemotherapy was prepared so it was early evening before it was administered. It was great to feel that the fightback against the illness was beginning. When you are first diagnosed a common reaction is to want to get started straight away on attacking it. Unfortunately, it does not quite work like that and, psychologically, waiting for treatment to begin is hard. This feeling was to be even stronger the next time I was ill when the lymphoma relapsed again.

The chemotherapy to be administered was a treatment called AVBD, named after the initials of the four drugs used: Adriamycin, Vinblastine, Bleomycin and Dacarbazine. Each drug was designed to attack the cancer cells at different stages of development. It was to be administered once every two weeks which did not seem too bad. I was told that it would make me feel tired for the first week and then I would pick up. However, blood counts would fall in the second week. Chemotherapy is a blunt instrument which destroys the cancer cells but destroys healthy cells as well.

There were also several possible side-effects. Adriamycin coloured my urine red or orange for several hours after treatment. This was not surprising since it looked like cherry lemonade as it went through the tube into the drip. This drug can also affect patients with heart problems although thankfully I was not in this category. Vinblastine caused pins and needles or numbness in the fingers and toes. This occurred for many months before it faded. Bleomycin can cause shivering and skin rashes and patients are advised to keep out of the sun for up to 24 hours after treatment to prevent skin rashes. In fact, I did not suffer from either of these side-effects. More frighteningly, Bleomycin can cause scarring of the lungs. This is one of those side-effects which is rare but there was no way of knowing whether it had affected me. Dacarbazine can cause pain in the veins if given into veins in the arm. Again, thankfully, this did not happen to me.

There were also general side-effects, common to many chemotherapy treatments. I could expect some hair loss and the destruction of blood cells. If red blood counts fell I would become more anaemic. A fall in white blood counts was of perhaps more concern because this would make me more prone to picking up infections.

There was some good news though. I was told that I could continue working if I felt up to it. This was a relief because when you are first diagnosed one of your main worries is 'Can I work?' and 'What about money?' because cancers do not clear up in a week or even a month. It is strange that I worried more about the wider consequences of the illness rather than what it might do to my body.

When the chemotherapy was first administered I did not know what to expect. In my case it was to be given intravenously although some forms of chemotherapy are given via tablets. There were three drugs administered through a syringe into the tube as well as an anti-sickness treatment. I remember two of these particularly for different reasons. As mentioned earlier there was the orange urine after Adriamycin was given while the Dacarbazine gave a tingling sensation in the backside about 30 seconds after it was administered. The Vinblastine was administered for 30 minutes through a drip from a bag which was covered up because it was light sensitive. The total time for administering the whole chemotherapy treatment each time was about 40 minutes.

The first chemotherapy treatment was finally administered on 25 August on Ward 10 in the early evening. Earlier, I had been moved into a bed in a different bay of Ward 10 after Sarah had grumbled on my behalf about the bad night's sleep I had experienced the night before. It was not certain at this stage that I would definitely be going home that day. So I was moved into a bay where there were other cancer sufferers rather than old men with strokes.

I met three others who were being treated for leukaemia. I was taken aback by how positive and jovial they were about their illnesses and how they were able to laugh about their setbacks and problems. One of them had had treatment for his leukaemia but had relapsed quickly so he could not have any more chemotherapy. He seemed so brave about it although I suspected that his prognosis was not good.

I realised that I was lucky; there were others who appeared to be worse off than me. I also realised that the only way to deal with this illness was to make light of it and laugh with others. We were all in it together. With one exception (the third time I was diagnosed), I have never met a cancer sufferer who was negative. You have to be positive otherwise you would just give up.

CHAPTER 6
Ups and Downs

Coming home was a good feeling in that I felt I was now fighting back and that everything was going to be fine. It was the final week of the summer holiday, which had obviously been ruined. However, it was warm and sunny so we sat in the garden, playing with Dominic, feeling that everything was going to be okay. This was reinforced when, one week later, blood tests revealed that the kidneys were working normally after just one treatment which was excellent news.

I then prepared to return to work. Firstly, I had to let my Headmaster, Robert Court, know of this illness because allowances would need to be made. He was shocked, along with my line manager Eric and the Deputy Head. It was also a huge shock for John Turner, my new assistant colleague, who was beginning his first term at the school although he was an experienced teacher. The reaction was what I expected from Birkdale School. Being a school with a deep Christian ethos they relieved me of as many duties as possible, such as being a form tutor. I was able to work through the whole term up to December although there were times when I went home early, feeling tired.

I soon developed a routine. Treatment was on a Friday, every two weeks. At first I did not feel too bad on the Saturday and we usually went out for tea to our favourite pub. It was important to keep family life as normal as possible. However by Sunday my taste buds seemed strange with most food tasting like cardboard! I did not enjoy Sunday lunch after a chemotherapy day - and Sarah cooks a wonderful Sunday lunch. I also needed to take my anti-sickness tablets for a few days after chemotherapy.

I then tried to go to work on the Monday but found I was very tired so eventually the school allowed me to stay at home on Mondays after chemotherapy. Eventually I became used to this pattern and learned to plan not to do anything too strenuous around the time when chemotherapy was administered. I was pleased that I managed to cope well at school up to half-term in October 2001. At home we managed to keep life as normal as it could be and at half-term we were able to take Dominic to the local fair and the illuminations at Matlock in Derbyshire. In November we were able to take him to a bonfire and fireworks.

However, not everything was perfect during this period. I had to have a blood transfusion in September as chemotherapy reduced the number of red blood cells. I became anaemic and was sent to Ward 10 as a day case which was the first time I met Elaine, a senior nurse. She was not the first nurse or doctor to have great difficulty in finding my veins. The transfused blood had to be dripped in through a cannula. That morning, perhaps because it was a Monday, Elaine managed to insert it into a small vein. After a while the blood seeped into the skin. I noticed that my arm was swelling up and when I pointed this out to Elaine alarm bells started ringing. She whipped out the cannula and wrapped bandages around to limit the bruising on the arm. There was a large area of bruising up my arm from my fingers to the elbow which took weeks to disappear. Elaine was a very kind and caring nurse and it was not her fault but she felt guilty about it for weeks afterwards. She would avoid my veins and ask someone else to insert the cannula. Whenever I see her today we still make a joke about it.

Another event in September was the sudden loss of hair which seemed to start happening after only one treatment. Upon washing my hair in the shower I looked in horror as clumps came away on the towel. Thin patches started appearing in my hair and I made two decisions before it was too late. One of these was to obtain a wig. Being a teacher I did not feel it appropriate to be without hair. Although my Headmaster indicated that it was fine to wear a cap around school I did not feel that it was professional: appearance is very important as a teacher. Also there was the thought of my head becoming cold as winter approached. I know that some men at that time chose to have their heads shaved but then that was their choice and if they wanted a cold head they could have one! The second decision was to have a new passport photograph taken before my hair disappeared. I was determined to get well and travel again.

I was given a voucher by the hospital to obtain a wig on the NHS. I found a wonderful hairdresser in Mansfield who sorted me out with a good wig which was then finished off by our hairdresser friend, Karen. At least I had been warned about my hair.

I was given an unexpected surprise when, after my second treatment, Kate, the other senior nurse, informed me that I was going to start GCSF injections. These are also called Neupogen syringes and contain a drug called Filgrastim. This stimulates the bone marrow in the body to produce more white blood cells to help replace those destroyed by chemotherapy. The bone marrow is 'the factory' where red and white blood cells are produced and, as discussed in the previous chapter, is suppressed during treatment.

The injections were to be administered into the stomach and the good news was that I would be able to do this myself. Kate took me into a side room and guided me through the process. It was not quite as bad as it sounded because it entailed finding the fleshy part of the stomach around the abdomen and there was plenty of that on me! Giving myself these injections became a way of life as it does for sufferers of diabetes.

This routine continued and we had a fairly normal life. This made it easier to deal with. I was also able to drive myself down to Derby for tests and chemotherapy which relieved the pressure on Sarah who was still receiving injections for her chronic fatigue. Although when it was chemotherapy day on a Friday, Sarah told me that I looked like an old man of ninety by the evening. Such compliments give you such a boost during treatment!

It was only in November that life became more of a struggle. Up to that point Sarah was amazed by my strength; that I had managed to hold down a full-time job and endure the treatment. She thought that I was very brave.

In November I seemed to develop a lot of catarrh and I pushed myself hard at school during what is a very important and busy time. There were tests for the Lower Sixth and various parents' evenings, including a Sixth Form recruitment evening which, as a Head of Department, was very crucial. I always believed that I would get better and so it was important that the future of the department was secured through maintaining numbers of students.

During this period I lost my voice and my cough seemed to come back. With hindsight, I should have taken some sick leave from work until I felt recharged. However, I worked until the end of term which I thought was a great achievement. It showed that chemotherapy need not wreck your life if you have a positive attitude. However, I was very tired. I remember on the last day of term falling asleep in the staffroom. Pushing myself so much was now bringing a price to pay.

On 7 December 2001 when I went to the hospital for my next chemotherapy session my white blood count was 11. This might not seem anything extraordinary because a minimum measure of 3 was required for chemotherapy to be given and the normal range for an adult is 4 to 11. However, I was puzzled because the GCSF injections normally boosted up the white counts to levels as high as 20-30. Chemotherapy was subsequently given but I did not realise at the time that this was to be my final dose of the AVBD chemotherapy.

When Christmas arrived I was tired and started to feel generally ill. I guessed that an infection had developed and if your white blood count is low you have little to fight it. There was a clear rule from the hospital that such symptoms were to be reported. My next chemotherapy treatment was due on 21 December. I discussed this with Sarah and agreed that I would ask Dr Grant for a postponement so that I could enjoy my Christmas food and would not be too tired. I then did something very unwise. I sensed that I had a temperature and knew that there was a danger of being admitted to Ward 10 if it was detected. I took two paracetamols before going to the hospital. I desperately wanted to avoid being admitted to hospital over Christmas, especially with a four-year-old son.

When I mentioned postponement to Dr Grant she agreed, stating that she did not think it would have any detrimental effect. I did mention the cough and that I had brought up some green phlegm so she prescribed some antibiotics which I took over Christmas and they seemed to make me feel better. Christmas Day was quite enjoyable except I developed a nasty ulcer on my tongue which was like having a large hole in the tongue. On Boxing Day I could hardly eat anything because of the pain I was in.

My next chemotherapy was due on 28 December. I had completed the antibiotics and started to feel ill again that morning. Kate took my blood test and stated that I would not have to wait too long for my chemotherapy because they were not too busy. Normally I went home after blood tests, telephoned for the results and came back in the afternoon for treatment.

I was not totally surprised when Kate informed me that I would not be having chemotherapy because my white blood count was only 1.9. She then took my temperature which was 37.7°C. I was then informed that I was to be admitted to Ward 10. I informed Dr Grant that I needed to drive home first. She was not happy but could not really stop me. I was told to come straight back. It was a shock to be admitted but I felt so ill I did not resist this time. As with the previous summer, I was concerned as to how it would affect Sarah. She called my mother and father down to help her with Dominic.

That night in hospital my temperature reached 39°C. Doctors were taking blood tests in the middle of the night and I was then put on antibiotic drips once every four hours. I was informed that it would take few days for things to improve. One unfortunate consequence of this was that I was to be in hospital on New Year's Eve. It was terrible to hear celebrations at midnight. I just turned over and went to sleep. The worst thing was that very near the hospital was the Florence Nightingale pub. The other patients and I did talk about tying the bedsheets together and escaping out of the window down to the pub! However, we thought better of it. One consolation was that one of the nurses brought a bottle of whisky round with late night hot drinks, but since I was on antibiotic drips it was not a good idea to have alcohol no matter how much I felt like it! However I was tempted because the 'hole' in my tongue had worsened. It was now a severe ulcer due to my very low white blood count. I was given antiseptic paste but maybe alcohol might have numbed it better!

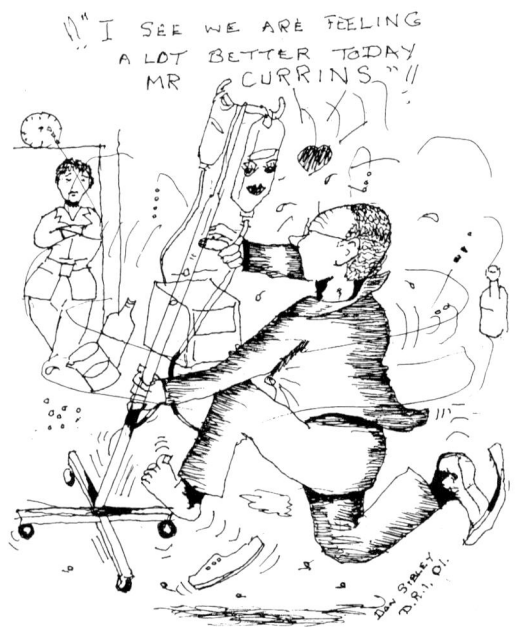

Although I was demoralised by another spell in hospital I had been warned that infections can develop with chemotherapy and since the bone marrow (and hence the immune system) is suppressed the body cannot fight these without assistance. It was also a difficult week for Sarah for visiting because the weather was freezing. In fact, it was the coldest week of the winter; not that I noticed it in the tropical confines of Ward 10. However, it was not a boring week, with good company in the bay. I met some interesting characters. Gerry in the next bed was suffering from blood clots on the chest. There was Don who kindly produced the cartoon depicting my stay in Ward 10 over the New Year. He was being treated with a chest problem. He summed up my frustration with being hooked up to drips. We had some laughs together which made the stay more bearable.

There were other amusing moments. One of these was when an Asian patient was admitted with a severe epileptic attack. As he recovered his family brought in some home-made onion bhargees. He had too many and offered them round the bay. I could tell they were very spicy as there was a bout of coughing around the bay! Unfortunately, I had to decline because I still had the 'hole' in my tongue and I would have leapt through the ceiling! It was very frustrating because I normally love Indian food. I had to smile on another day when his friend smuggled some cans of beer into the bay under the nose of Sister, and there was a party in the corner.

Eventually I was allowed home on 2 January. The hospital had conducted a bone marrow biopsy while I was on the ward to assess what progress had been made before the chemotherapy had gone wrong. They wanted to keep me in the ward a little longer but Sarah needed me at home desperately. The problem was that my white blood counts were only recovering very slowly and this seemed to be a cause for concern.

I also realised that I would not be returning to school after the Christmas holiday. Sarah informed Birkdale that we did not know at this stage when I would return. In fact, it was to be just over half a term before I could do so.

When I returned home I then finally had time to think. I started to worry about what would happen next. Chemotherapy had been suspended because of the seriousness of the infection. Would the illness creep back? Had I had enough treatment?

I returned to clinic on 8 January 2002 to see Dr McKernan. She was a Consultant I had seen around the ward but Dr Grant had seemed to be in charge. Dr McKernan now seemed to be in charge of my case as Dr Grant appeared not to be there any more. I awaited the bone marrow result. She informed Sarah and I that there was some uncertainty about the bone marrow and the sample was being sent off to Nottingham City Hospital for another opinion. This was not very comforting but one encouraging fact was that I had started to feel quite well and my kidney function was fine. I was told to return to clinic in one week's time on 15 January.

January 15 came and it was a significant day. Sarah had gone to college for her GCSE Maths class. As part of maintaining normal life I insisted that she continued with her studying. When I was getting dressed I noticed some tenderness in my groin. When I felt the particular area there appeared to be a lump. I was horrified because there had never been any lumps in the groin area before. I remembered that Dr Thomas had always felt the groin area very thoroughly in past check-ups and there had never been anything.

It seemed a weird coincidence that on the morning I was going to clinic I had noticed this. I met Sarah from college and, as we went down to Derby, I found it hard how to tell her what I had discovered. Sarah tried to reassure me but I could tell she was worried by the look on her face. Afterwards Sarah told me that her stomach was churning. She was horrified that it might now be a worse outcome. Up to then she expected me to be cured.

At clinic Dr McKernan informed us that the bone marrow results were still inconclusive. They needed more time to consider opinions. In the meantime there were no plans to resume chemotherapy. This was a blow because waiting for results is awful. When you do not receive anything conclusive it prolongs the agony.

I then reported the lump in the groin. She examined it and then stated that it would be removed for a biopsy in the next week. She then discussed a bone marrow cross-match and asked if I had any brothers or sisters. I do have two brothers living in Hull. Dr McKernan wanted to blood test them and me to assess whether they were a cross-match in the event that a bone marrow transplant might be needed.

My CT scan was booked in for 17 January, which seemed to be a significant date for me once again. This was to assess if the stomach lymph nodes had reduced in size. On 21 January the cross-match blood tests were conducted. Two days later I had the biopsy operation to remove the lump in the groin.

Since December it had all seemed like bad news. However, on the morning of the 23rd Alan Bryan came to see me on the ward before my operation. That day had started bleakly; I had to report early to a surgical ward and then there had been no bed. Eventually, I was found a bed on an optical ward which was very nice and modern. At last Alan had some good news for me. He told me that the CT scan had revealed that the stomach lymph nodes had reduced in size more than might have been expected for the amount of chemotherapy I had received - only two-thirds of the treatment had been completed before the infection. This gave me great hope.

Even so, the day was full of tension. Since the previous midnight my status had been nil by mouth and it was nearly 4.30 p.m. before I was taken to theatre. Just to add to the tension, Sarah phoned me at the hospital and told me that her father had been admitted to hospital with heart problems. Poor Sarah did not know which way to turn. That day she had received a telephone call from her worried mother saying that her elderly father had gone out earlier and had not returned. Sarah had to telephone the local hospital to find out what had happened to her father. She found out he was in Casualty and no-one had told her mother. However, on a topsy-turvy day she had received news earlier that day from college that her score in a mathematics examination had been 100%.

When I finally arrived at the theatre the anaesthetist was very pleasant but she was concerned about my infamous veins, so I was given gas initially. This brought back horrible memories of visiting the school clinic dentist to have three teeth out when I was five years old. It is strange how feelings of many years ago can be revived.

However, this time I knew little about it and my next experience was waking up with a huge patch on my groin. This area was also very sore but my main concern was having something to eat and drink. Unfortunately, I had missed my meal but a nurse brought me some sandwiches which I devoured in a very short time. I had to stay in the ward for one night because the operation had been so late but I was the only patient in the bay and it was very pleasant.

The weeks following my arrival home again were a waiting game. My next appointment at clinic was 5 February. This proved to be an unhappy day. Firstly, we had a late appointment slot at 12.00. It was a long wait and the tension builds all the time, especially when you are awaiting biopsy results. There was also still the matter of the bone marrow result where there had been some uncertainty. The tension was heightened because Dominic had to be picked up from school which meant leaving Derby no later than 2.30 p.m. Whilst waiting, we saw a friend of ours, Sid Miles, from the Baptist Church in Swanwick. They had been praying for me since I relapsed but then Sid, who was a deacon of the church, was himself diagnosed with Non-Hodgkin's Lymphoma. He had come to clinic himself that day for a check-up during his chemotherapy and appeared to be doing quite well. That day he was accompanied by Rev. Roy Plant, a retired Baptist minister, who was to give me support during my third relapse. It helped to have someone to chat to because waiting rooms for these clinics can be filled with tension. Everyone knows that you are not there with a trivial illness.

We were finally seen at 2.25 p.m. and could afford no more than five to ten minutes. This was really difficult because you cannot be looking at the clock when you are receiving such information. Dr McKernan had mixed results. Firstly, the good news was that the bone marrow was clear of the disease. However, they thought that the lump in the groin revealed a different type of Hodgkin's Disease called Nodular Sclerosis. This was more common than the Lymphocyte Predominant type it had previously been.

The bad news was that it would be more difficult to cure. We were informed that it would require a stem cell transplant which would involve intensive chemotherapy and several hospital stays. We were stunned. However, there was a glimmer of hope. Dr McKernan stated that there was still a 10% chance it could still be Lymphocyte Predominant. This was more easily curable and would involve using a relatively new drug called Mabthera which would not have the nasty side-effects of conventional chemotherapy. The lump was now with Nottingham City Hospital for a second opinion. We should know in one week when Alan would ring me.

This was probably the lowest point for Sarah and I. We became resigned to a stem cell transplant but still hoped and prayed that it would not come to this. In fact there was a great deal of prayer going on: prayer meetings were frequent during this period both at the local Baptist church and at Birkdale School. Sarah later told me that at this point she was very worried about what the future held. At times she felt quite numb.

One week went by and Alan did not contact me with the result. When Sarah went for her injections for chronic fatigue Dr Skidmore told Sarah that identifying cancer cells was like identifying birds in the sky from a distance. We realised that it must therefore not be clear cut and it would be better that they took their time to gain a correct diagnosis.

I wondered if I should contact Alan but then, although I desperately wanted to know, I dared not pick up the telephone. As each day went by the tension in the house grew. I kept telling myself that I did actually feel a great deal better, which had to be a good sign. Since Christmas my blood counts had recovered and I actually felt ready to return to work. On 14 February we decided to book a meal out for Valentine's Day. I felt very well and life seemed normal. My hair was growing back again. Even so, we both knew there was unfinished business.

On Friday 15 February we both decided that it had to be faced. I telephoned Alan who informed me that there was no result yet but that I should ring again at 4.30 that afternoon; even then however there was no guarantee of a result from Nottingham City Hospital. In the afternoon Sarah had to go out because she could not stand the tension any longer. I telephoned again at 4.30 and Alan informed me that there was still no result but that Dr McKernan was just walking in so if she knew anything they would phone back quickly. Fifteen minutes later it was Dr McKernan herself who phoned back. She had good news. Nottingham City Hospital Consultant Dr Andy Haynes had decided that the lump in the groin was still Lymphocyte Predominant. Dr Haynes was and still is one of the top specialists for lymphoma cancers and he was to later take full control of my treatment when I relapsed for the third time.

Thankfully, it was not to be intensive chemotherapy or a stem cell transplant. Instead, I was to receive four sessions of a drug called Mabthera. This is an expensive drug which stimulates the body's immune system to attack the cancer cells and destroy them. It was very good news because it would not affect the blood cells and my hair would not fall out again. Sarah and I hugged each other.

At this point I decided to seek a return to school as soon as possible and went back on 25 February after an absence of seven weeks. When treatment began the drug was administered by intravenous drip for five hours each session. It was a painless experience apart from the usual difficulty of finding veins in my arms - a problem which had intensified as a result of the AVBD chemotherapy. At the end of the four weeks I was to have a bone marrow biopsy and a CT scan to assess whether the drug treatment had been successful. I was warned that if this had not worked it would mean the stem cell transplant after all.

The biopsy was on 25 March which I felt was a good omen because it was the 20th anniversary of my great-grandmother's death. I had been very close to her when she was alive and felt she still was looking over me. As usual I had the sedative for the biopsy. When I came round I seemed unsteady on my feet. It felt as if I had had several drinks. Our friend Sid Miles was unfortunately in Ward 10 that day. Sarah and I went to see him but I probably did not make much sense! We were later saddened to hear of his death on 29 March which was Good Friday. Sid was not afraid of death but it was still hard when he seemed so well in February. He was a good Christian man and it seemed poignant that he died that day. We shall always be grateful to him, his wife Margaret and the Baptist Church in general for their support.

The CT scan was on 11 April, our wedding anniversary. Again, I thought that it was a good omen. Finally, I was to attend clinic on 16 April to receive the results. Again, this seemed like another positive omen because it was Dominic's fifth birthday. It was a lovely sunny spring morning. I took Dominic to school and remember *'Flowers in the Window'* by Travis was playing on the radio. It is a very cheerful tune and it seemed to signal a happy, optimistic morning. I had a good feeling as I attended clinic.

When Dr McKernan came in to see me she was smiling. The scan results were good because the stomach lymph nodes had reduced in size considerably. What was left was believed to be scar tissue. The bone marrow was also clear; they would see me in three months time. I was in remission although doctors never actually tell you this; it is simply implied. That evening we went out as a family for a celebratory meal on Dominic's birthday. We could now get our lives back on track again. Sarah was now feeling more optimistic about the future. I was elated though deep down I knew I was wondering whether I had in fact seen the last of the disease.

CHAPTER 7
Relapse

In the months following April 2002 I had wonderful health. My blood counts were very healthy and I had a great deal of energy. I was on three-monthly check-ups and these continued to be fine except for a scare in the September when an enzyme value called LDH went up, suggesting a lymphoma. I did not know what this meant but thankfully a CT scan revealed that everything was still clear and the enzyme value returned to normal.

Stability returned to the Business Studies department at school and I found that I was able to slot back into everything fairly easily. I was determined to make up for the stagnant period in my life.

We had a very happy summer - a complete contrast to 2001. There were four holidays in the period from July 2002 to May 2003. We went to Majorca in July 2002, our first holiday since the treatment ended. This was followed by Paris in August including a visit to EuroDisney. In January 2003 we went to Lanzarote and then in May travelled to Majorca again. These were wonderful holidays and they were followed by a happy autumn when my brother, Martin, married Debbie in October. It was wonderful to have a wedding in the family after all that had happened. It was also wonderful for me to be Best Man for him. Sarah did a reading in church and Dominic was a page-boy. In my speech I mentioned how, in marriage, love can overcome anything including serious illness. For Sarah and I that was certainly the case.

An exciting and successful academic year at Birkdale School then followed between 2002 and 2003. The department expanded as numbers grew. There was also success in extracurricular areas. The school Young Enterprise companies won eight trophies in 2003 and reached the Yorkshire and Humber Regional Final at the McAlpine Stadium in Huddersfield on 19 June.

There were other memorable events. On 18 March I met Eric Clapton, who had come to Birkdale School to perform 'An Audience with Eric Clapton'. I had the great pleasure of teaching Eric's daughter and he wanted to meet all of her subject tutors for a mini parents' evening after the show.

I also met Paul Hudson, the BBC Look North Weather presenter at an Institute of Directors Awards lunch. I was being presented with the runner-up prize in the tutor category of an export competition.

Spring of 2003 thus seemed to be a 'golden' period of personal and departmental success. Life was good and the traumas of 2001 seemed to have been left far behind. I felt we were entering a better period of our lives and my career was on an upward trend. However, life has a habit of kicking you in the teeth when you least expect it.

As early as January 2003, after we returned from Lanzarote, a slight shadow started to appear on the horizon. One night, after having a bath, I noticed a small lump in the groin on the spot where the lymph node had been removed the previous January. I was not over-concerned because I had noticed back then that the area was raised after the operation, which I assumed to be scar tissue. Life was going so well with exciting developments at school that I did not want any disruption. On 28 January I went for my check-up and the Registrar routinely checked the groin area. She did not seem concerned by anything so I thought no more about it at that time.

In April I was slightly concerned when my red blood count dropped slightly to 13.9. It had been running at between 14.7 to 14.9 on the previous check-ups which were near the top of the scale. I was told not to worry because it was still well above the minimum normal value of 11.5 and such a drop was insignificant. Everything seemed fine although I was still concerned by the raised area in the groin, although the doctor still did not seem to notice anything after examining that area.

In July I started to have some suspicions of possible trouble ahead. At the latest check-up the Registrar did express concern about something in the left groin; but the blood tests were all fine and so she decided not to act at this stage. My red blood count had not fallen any more, remaining at 13.9, which also gave me some encouragement. I was then informed that there would be a routine CT scan before the next clinic check-up and this began a summer of anxiety.

I normally looked forward to the summer holiday and it had been such a successful year at school I should have been feeling a warm glow of satisfaction. Moreover, since the student numbers had expanded in my department we had appointed a third (part-time) teacher for September. The future should have been looking bright. However, there was a feeling of fear.

During the summer holiday I felt depressed although there was no obvious reason for this. The weather was fabulous and we saw old friends. However, I found that minor issues began to irritate me and I became less tolerant when little things went wrong. I started developing feelings of not wanting to go back to school in September. This was strange after one of the most successful periods in my teaching career. Perhaps I was afraid that I could not live up to that standard again. No; it was more than that, though at that point I did not realise why I was experiencing such feelings.

There were some positives, too. For example, I raised some money from car boot sales to buy a CD radio unit for the Haematology Day Case unit at the Derbyshire Royal Infirmary. They were delighted with this though I remarked that I hoped that I would never need to get direct benefit from it myself. I was to regret these comments later on.

A significant date for me was 22 August 2003. I woke up with some sciatic pain down my right leg. I had not experienced this since 1988 when I dislodged a joint in my back and almost prolapsed a disc.

That weekend we had planned a busy time. On 23rd August we visited our friends in Preston and then on the 24th went to Hull to my parents for a few days. I do not know how but my mother is very perceptive when it comes to illness in the family. She kept asking if there was something that I wasn't telling her. I did have fear but at this stage did not realise what was to come. Later on, when I relapsed, my mother told me that she just knew that I was not well. Back in 2001 when Hodgkin's first returned my mother was not surprised. She thought that I had looked tired for a few years.

However, it was obvious that my health was not at its best once again. Whilst in Hull I developed conjunctivitis in one eye and had to obtain a prescription for some eye drops.

Upon returning home I decorated our bedroom and found it a real struggle. I felt under pressure to do this once Dominic had returned to school. It is difficult to decorate with a six-year-old around. However I did not feel physically or mentally that I wanted to do the job.

I then developed a chest infection at the beginning of September which required some antibiotics and the sciatica seemed worse after the decorating. I had to miss a practical training day held on the first day of term at Edale in Derbyshire

I managed to return to work the next day but was struggling with the sciatica. I went to an osteopath who said that I had prolapsed the disc which had given me trouble in 1988. I also felt very tired and noticed after three weeks of the new term that I was finding it difficult to climb up the stairs to my classroom. I also found that during lessons I was going into the office for small drinks of water. These were ominous signs as I approached the CT scan and clinic check-up, although at the time I did not realise that the lymphoma was returning.

I had my CT scan on 25 September and went for my routine blood tests on 10 October. It was the day of the Birkdale 'whole school' photograph and I was very concerned to have my blood tests completed quickly and to arrive at school in time for the photograph. Perhaps deep down I knew it would be my final appearance in such a photograph.

On the evening of 10 October there was a staff social evening at school which Sarah and I attended. It was very enjoyable but I felt exhausted even though it was a Friday. I always felt tired on Fridays but found the energy to enjoy the event. I did not realise what was to come in the very near future.

During the weekend of 11-12 October I felt gloomy. I did not feel at all optimistic this time about my check-up. I expected problems although I did not share these feelings with Sarah. However my Deputy Head, Andrew Johnson, realised that I was not well.

Two weeks before clinic our new part-time member of staff suddenly resigned after a supper evening at the Head Master's house, a traditional event to welcome new staff. I am sure it was not the excellent food which caused her to resign! A number of factors had built up to her decision but I had been too wrapped up with my health to really notice. Trying to cover her lessons, on top of my other worries, caused enormous additional stress.

On Monday 13 October I indicated to Andrew that I was not too optimistic but I did not realise then that the day was to be the last of my teaching career.

Tuesday 14 October duly dawned. I drove down to Derby on my own as I had on previous check-ups. My appointment time was 10.00 a.m. but I began to feel that something was not right when other patients arrived after me and then were seen before me. In fact, I seemed to be the final patient to be seen, over an hour after my appointment time.

When I was finally called into the waiting cubicle I could hear a discussion in the office next door and when I heard the comment; 'why has it returned so extensively?', I knew that the news would be bad. Eventually, Alan Bryan, whom I knew well, came out with a Registrar I had never seen before. Alan informed me that it was indeed not good news this time. The CT scan had revealed swollen stomach lymph nodes again and there were three suspicious lumps in the groin. Furthermore the blood test results were abnormal. The level of calcium salts was up again and my red blood count had fallen to 10 so I was anaemic again. They needed to admit me to Ward 10 that afternoon.

I simply sat there feeling as if my world had collapsed. It felt like the end of my life. I felt very angry at first and took it out on Alan and the Registrar. I wanted to blame someone but it was not their fault.

I left the building in a daze. I always rang Sarah when I left the hospital building and usually everything was fine. I could scarcely pick up the mobile phone to tell Sarah this time. I could hardly speak for tears. Then I had to return home to pack a bag. Instead of returning to school that afternoon I was to be admitted to Ward 10, a place I was all too familiar with. I did not know what the future would hold but I knew it would be a long road ahead.

All of this was once again a huge shock to Sarah and she felt numb once again. Although I had had my suspicions that all was not going to be well I did not discuss it with Sarah. She had sensed my feelings of depression after the July clinic check-up but did not think the disease was returning.

However Sarah told me that she had a dream in June and woke up in a hot sweat. Someone had spoken to her and said, 'Russell's going to be ill again. He will need a stem cell transplant.' Sarah did not know who it was, perhaps it was a message from God? She did not want to believe it at the time. In late summer she was spoken to in a dream in the same way. Again, she did not want to believe it although it did play on her mind this time. However, Sarah was still stunned when I told her the news.

Sarah later told me in November she was spoken to again in the same way and told that, 'for sure Russell will be having a stem cell transplant'. My fate was apparently sealed.

CHAPTER 8
Transformation

As I lay in the bed in Ward 10 again there was a strong sense of déjà vu. The dreaded cannula was inserted into the vein in my hand and I was put on saline drips to re-hydrate my body. Alan came to speak to me and I apologised for my outburst in the morning. He told me he gets such reactions quite often when patients are told bad news. After he left my first thoughts were about the chaos that my absence would cause at Birkdale School. I spent two hours preparing a list of tasks for John Turner, my colleague, who would now be running the department in my absence. I felt very sorry for him because he would be faced with an increased work load which he did not really want.

I also felt sorry for my pupils to whom I had said the previous week that I thought my check-up would be fine, with no problems. I also felt for poor Sarah and Dominic who would have to suffer in coping without me once again. Sarah had hoped upon hope that everything would be all right and, even if it had not been, believed that things would not be too bad. However when I told her the news she felt that our lives had changed in a 'flash'. Her feelings were, 'Oh, what a long road ahead, particularly with winter approaching'. She braced herself for what was to come. It is strange that when diagnosed with a relapse you tend not to think of yourself. Cancer affects a much wider range of people than just the individual patient.

Despite all of these concerns I felt a strange sense of relief. There were two aspects to this. Firstly, I had been concerned for a while that my health was not quite right and now the worst was known I could start fighting back again.

Secondly, it had been an unhappy start to the school term because of my struggle with the prolapsed disc and the sudden departure of a member of staff. It was undeniably a relief, in my run-down state, not to have to struggle on and hold the department together although I felt bad about leaving John with this task.

I also began to realise that there might be a new role in life for me. When I returned to Ward 10 I was the youngest patient, except for Matthew, who was 18 years old. He had leukaemia and was scared that he was going to die. He was only the age of some of my Upper Sixth pupils and this made me realise that there were still other people worse off than myself. I found myself at ease at being able to talk to patients such as Matthew and I realised I had the ability to inject some positive hope. This role would emerge again during my next stay in hospital when I was to meet Greg.

There certainly were other patients worse off than me. I felt very sad for elderly men who had experienced strokes. One of these was 88 years old and had a very sound mind. He was very frustrated about what had happened. Another was so poorly that he could barely reach full consciousness. There were others with chest problems and some of these coughed a great deal at night and kept me awake. I did not feel annoyance at this but great pity. I had every determination to get well again but it would be more of a struggle for many of my fellow patients.

I spent four days in Ward 10. Whilst there I had another bone marrow biopsy, something I dreaded. I knew what the result would show. There was also a CT scan and an operation to remove the largest lump in the groin which I suspected to be scar tissue. This took place on Friday 17 October, the anniversary of the date Sarah and I first met in 1985. We would normally have celebrated with a meal at a decent restaurant in the evening and this was to be the first year that it was not going to happen.

I have memories of this operation because this time I was given a local anaesthetic with a sedative to calm me. This was described as the 'gin and tonic' and was designed to ensure that I would not remember too much even though I would be awake. I cannot remember the surgeon cutting me open and removing the lump but I do remember seeing the theatre nurses sewing me up through a reflective 'mirror' on the ceiling. I was then shown the lump in a jar; it looked grey. However, because of the sedative, I had a feeling of peace; whatever the surgeon had done, I would not have cared.

It was a good feeling when it was over but I felt very sore afterwards. I then attended as a day case for the calcium salts to be checked. These levels had now come down. I also had a date to attend clinic on 28 October for the biopsy results. The one fact I felt sure about was that it was to be more chemotherapy and Alan hinted that it would probably mean a stem cell transplant since the cancer had relapsed so quickly.

I had made two important decisions whilst in Ward 10. Since I had relapsed so rapidly I began to ask myself whether it was the stress and pace of the job which had caused it. Sarah blamed my job and the commuting in 2001 for my illness because it followed an unhappy period of stress. I now shared her belief and did not need much persuading about what to do about it. Sarah was determined that I was not going to return to teaching and I was not going to argue. I decided to seek medical retirement but at this stage I decided to keep the decision just between Sarah and I. The other important decision was to write this book. I wanted to give hope to future cancer sufferers and to raise some funds for cancer charities from the proceeds. I decided I would also aim to do some voluntary work, perhaps talking to patients to attempt to lift their spirits. It is important to establish a positive attitude especially at the beginning of that long, dark tunnel when you are first diagnosed. I was determined that some good should come out of this latest setback in my life.

Back at home the following week I obtained advice from my trade union representative about medical retirement and the appropriate forms. Although my mind was pretty much made up, I decided not to discuss this with Birkdale School yet nor actually to begin the process in case I might change my mind. It was a big decision to make after all.

By now it was half-term, my calcium salts remained steady and I felt reasonably well. We took Dominic to the local fair and attempted to have as normal a half-term holiday as possible. On 28 October Sarah and I attended clinic to hear the results of the biopsy. To our surprise, the lump which had been removed turned out to be merely dead tissue but, as expected, the disease was back in the bone marrow with half the marrow being affected. At this stage it was thought to be a return of Hodgkin's Disease. However there was a great feeling of anti-climax. When you attend clinics to receive news it is sometimes as bad to be given inconclusive news as it is to receive bad news. The agony of not knowing what was wrong was to go on.

The really bad news was that I needed another biopsy operation. Dr McKernan wanted to avoid a repeat of the previous result and stated that there would be an ultrasound and aspiration test on the largest remaining lump in the groin to establish if it was an active lymphoma and not just dead tissue. The biopsy operation would follow. We presumed that this would all happen with some urgency. However, there was no ultrasound appointment for two weeks because the necessary doctor was on holiday. In the meantime events took a nose-dive.

On Monday 3 November I went for a blood test; my calcium salt levels had risen again to 2.98 (the normal upper range is 2.54). On Wednesday 5th I received a telephone call from Alan to come down to the Day Case Unit at Derby immediately for some treatment.

I was determined not to be admitted to Ward 10 again because I wanted to take Dominic to a bonfire and fireworks that evening. When I arrived at the Day Case Unit my blood was tested again and the level of calcium salts had risen to 3.3. Normally I should have been admitted to the ward because of the danger of renal failure but I pleaded with the doctor and instead he prescribed a steroid drug which would be administered intravenously. This was designed to break up the calcium salts. I was allowed home and they arranged to see me again the following Monday.

When I was tested again my calcium salt level had jumped up to 3.88 which was dangerously high and as a result I was given a stronger steroid drug at the Day Case Unit. Alan really wanted to admit me to Ward 10 but I pleaded to be allowed home because in that particular week Sarah felt very poorly with flu and we had no family support nearby. I told him I felt fine but he always knew I was putting on an act to stay out of hospital.

This day was significant, not particularly because of the calcium salts but because it was the day I first came across Greg. This arose because the drug I was given took a long time to drip into the vein. When the Day Case Unit closed at 4.30 p.m. I was moved to Ward 10 to complete it. I was given a chair next to a bed near the window. In the bed on the right-hand side I could hear a young man telling a nurse that he had been given some bad news. Apart from saying hello I did not discuss it with him because I did not hear everything in the conversation. This young man was Greg, who had Non-Hodgkin's Lymphoma. We were to become friends and would support each other through the coming months.

After my treatment was completed that day I went home and was booked to return to clinic the next day. When I attended clinic Alan and a new Registrar called Addy wanted to admit me to Ward 10 that morning because of the dangerously high level of calcium salts. I again resisted because Sarah was still poorly. In the end, a compromise was reached. I agreed to go up to Ward 10 to have some more treatment but I was to be allowed home in the evening. I then agreed to return the next day when I would be admitted.

By coincidence, I also had my ultrasound appointment that same morning of 11 November. The lumps were very visible on the scan. There was a large one and a smaller one underneath it. The ultrasound doctor stated that it looked like an active lymphoma but there needed to be an aspiration test to be absolutely certain. He aimed to arrange this for the next day.

After the ultrasound examination I made my way up to Ward 10. I was given the drug to deal with the calcium salts. Once again a cannula was inserted into my hand and the drug was administered intravenously. By early evening it was finally completed and I was allowed to go home. However I did not feel at all well. I was dizzy and disorientated. I did not say anything to the nursing staff because I knew that I would not be allowed to drive home! The cannula was also left in my hand for the next day. It was carefully bandaged up so that I could drive.

I remember driving home feeling scared because I knew that I should not have been driving. It was dark and there seemed to be numerous headlights heading towards me. Anyway, I made it home safely and dived straight for the settee to lie down. There have been few occasions in my life when I have felt really scared but this was one of them. When I arrived home Sarah was horrified to see my ashen face and the state I was in.

On Wednesday 12 November I finally admitted defeat and packed a bag for Ward 10. Sarah drove me down to be admitted properly. I was a very sick man who had resisted hospital as long as possible. It was a relief now to be admitted.

When I arrived at Ward 10 it was not long before a porter came to take me for the aspiration test. There was a device attached to the ultrasound machine which injected a sharp needle into the suspect lump in the groin from which cells were extracted for examination.

Dr Robinson, who had conducted my first aspiration test in 1995, now tested these cells to assess if they were active. This was confirmed and a biopsy operation was needed to remove that lump. Things seemed to be happening very quickly; I was informed that the operation would take place the next day, 13 November.

I was given a local anaesthetic and the 'gin and tonic' once again. During this operation I seemed to be more alert and could actually feel the surgeon tugging at the lump which seemed to be deeper than the previous one which had been removed. I actually remember saying, 'this is hurting!' and subsequently more 'gin and tonic' was given. Afterwards it also seemed more sore than had been the case the last time. The next day, 14 November, I had another operation. This was to fit a Hickman Line into my chest - this would enable blood to be taken and treatments to be administered without the need for any further needles. I was not enthusiastic about having one but every doctor and nurse was having so many problems finding my veins that it was a relief that I would not have to be pierced with needles every time I received treatment.

The fitting was an operation in itself and I was given the 'gin and tonic' once again. However on this occasion I did not remember anything about the operation. I woke up with a tube with two valves sticking out of my chest with two lots of stitches.

Whilst in Ward 10 apart from the operations my calcium salt level had been falling and on Sunday 16th I was allowed home in the afternoon. This last stay in Ward 10 had certainly been interesting with a great deal of action. I had also found the company in the bay enjoyable. There were two men suffering respiratory problems, Gordon and Horace. They were very friendly and interesting to talk to. I had also been in the same bay as Greg who I had first met on the Monday. He was only 27 years old and was scared. He knew that he needed a bone marrow transplant eventually to cure his Non-Hodgkin's Lymphoma. He had been battling with a nasty lump in the neck since the previous May. Previous chemotherapy did not seem to be getting to grips with it. He was now to be given Mabthera. I was happily able to tell him how effective it had been for me in March 2002. I was able to talk to him and provide hope. I was able to tell him that if I had beaten this illness twice before, he could do it as well.

I also met Matthew again in another bay of Ward 10. He needed a bone marrow transplant and his brother was a perfect match but he was scared of dying and did not want the transplant. Again, I talked with him and later, his mother told me that he had gone ahead with it. I was beginning to realise that I might have a talent for helping lift fellow sufferers and that I might be able to pursue this as voluntary work. I did not find it difficult because I knew what it felt like to suffer.

After this latest spell in Ward 10 my blood was checked on the following Monday and Wednesday. On Friday 21st I was to receive the results of the biopsy. Dr McKernan and Alan called me into a side room to give me the news. I was told that the disease had transformed itself into Non-Hodgkin's Lymphoma. It was T-cell rich B. There are 20 different types of Non-Hodgkin's Lymphoma so it did not mean a great deal to me. However, I was given a booklet about it and it was interesting to see that the top possible cause was suppression of the immune system (immunosuppression). The literature suggests that the immune system fails to destroy cancer cells at an early stage. Research appears to suggest that Non-Hodgkin's Lymphoma tends to develop more often in patients who experience a reduction in the immune system for some reason.

Sarah later informed me from her knowledge of psychology that studies have shown that stress can cause the immune system to be suppressed. This suggested a link between stress and my illness. My mind was finally made up to seek medical retirement in earnest.

I was further told that chemotherapy was to begin on Monday 24 November. It was to be a four-day treatment called IVE. This was based on a regime of three drugs called Ifosfamide, Estoposide and Epirubicin. I am still unsure to this day where the 'V' came into it! These drugs were designed to attack the cancer at different stages of development as AVBD had done previously. It was also to prepare for a stem cell transplant. I would have this regime at least twice, eventually leading to a stem cell transplant. Inevitably, there would be the usual side-effects such as hair loss and bone marrow suppression leading to falling blood counts. There were other possible side effects which are described in the next chapter.

I was very calm about this even when told that it was now a high-grade lymphoma, i.e. more aggressive. I do not know why I was so calm. It was just a shock that it had transformed itself from Hodgkin's Disease to Non-Hodgkin's. I knew that the prognosis was not as good. However, battle had once again to commence.

CHAPTER 9
Dark Days and Hope

I was admitted to Ward 10 on Sunday 23 November 2003 to begin the first course of IVE chemotherapy. It was a great relief to be starting some treatment to fight back against the illness. It was particularly important because it would prevent the calcium salts building up again so the kidneys could function properly. When I entered Ward 10 it must have been one of the few times I had a smile on my face. Before I left home it had been very difficult. Sarah was finding it hard that I would be going into hospital for four nights at least. The final evening was a tearful one and she felt unable to drive me to hospital. Luckily, I asked a kind neighbour across the road who took me there instead. With any sort of cancer it is the emotional and physical strain suffered by the partner or spouse which many people fail to notice. The patient seems to receive all of the attention.

Sarah had originally said back in the October when I was first diagnosed that she could not cope but amazingly she had found great strength until this point. On Ward 10 another reason for a smile on my face was the allocation of a single room. Although I can sympathise with the suffering of other patients in a bay it is undoubtedly better in a single room because there is less noise and sleep is easier.

The IVE chemotherapy was to be dripped in over five days intravenously through the Hickman Line. However initially I was given saline drips to fully hydrate me to cope with the drugs. I was then delighted to discover that I was to be given Mabthera to begin the treatment. It was Mabthera which had been given to me in March 2002 and which had seemed to bring 18 months of wonderful health. After the Mabthera there was a selection of drugs given continuously day and night. As soon as one bag was completed another was set up. The pump was almost continually attached to me through the Hickman Line during this chemotherapy. It was a nuisance but it was worse when I had a tube attached to a cannula because movement of the arm was restricted and it hurt.

I came to name it my 'ball and chain'. I felt like a prisoner restrained by a tube instead of a handcuff. Everywhere the pump went, I went including the toilet and the bath. Sometimes I would be released, freedom felt wonderful!

There were various possible side effects associated with the main chemotherapy drugs. The drug Ifosfamide carried the risk of fits and going into a coma so I was given an anti-epileptic drug (Phenytoin) to combat this. Furthermore, Ifosfamide could cause bleeding in the bladder so every time I paid a visit to the toilet I had to fill up a jug with urine. I was given a further drug called Mensa to help prevent this effect. As the treatment went on visits to the toilet became more frequent. This disturbed my sleep on a number of occasions. The nurses had to check my jug of urine after each toilet visit and must have thought, 'Not another one!' It must have been one of the less pleasant aspects of nursing!

Epirubicin could cause heart failure, even in patients with no known heart problems. This was a drug I was familiar with from the AVBD regime. This was the drug which had made my urine go orange. Etoposide could cause low blood pressure whilst being given. Surprisingly, this did not affect me even though I normally had low blood pressure anyway. Low blood pressure is unusual for a teacher!

Thankfully, I did not have a fit or any heart failure! However, I did feel a little spaced out after four days of treatment. One day my vision seemed a little blurred but this passed. One positive aspect was a lack of sickness. I only felt a little nauseous on the last day of treatment. Thankfully, the anti-sickness drugs were very effective.

Sarah visited me every day and she wondered what state she would find me in as she too had been warned that I could lapse into a coma. Sarah visited me whenever possible. She even came after college on any Thursdays I was in hospital because she studied law in Derby on those evenings. As before, I wanted her to continue with her studies to keep her mind occupied. In fact, Sarah told me that keeping busy helped her through it all.

In the room I had my own TV and video. I asked Sarah to fetch me a selection of videos to pass the time. Boredom is one of the worse aspects of being in hospital, particularly when you are in a room on your own. You can lay for a long time without speaking to anyone. Sometimes I would visit Greg who was in another room during the same period. We would watch 'Match of the Day' videos together.

I used to hate the nights. I did not sleep well and would hear nurses chatting in the corridor. Also I was disturbed by the pump which dripped in the chemotherapy. I could hear the gurgling of the fluids going into my Hickman Line. When a chemotherapy bag was empty or the tube blocked the pump would bleep and wake me up. Then a nurse came in and the light went on.

I was always glad when it was 7 o'clock because it was not long to breakfast, then cleaners would appear so there was someone to talk to, followed by nurses who changed the beds everyday and would have a joke with you, then Sarah would appear in the morning to visit me. There would also be a visit from the team of doctors each day who would inform you of your progress. I looked forward to seeing the doctors particularly when Dr Maine came around. He was always light hearted and would make jokes.

Lunch was a high point. The food was very good. However afternoons were depressing especially after Sarah had gone because Dominic needed picking up from school. I used to watch TV, write some of the book or sleep. Then came teatime, again the food was good. Evenings were not so bad because at least there was plenty to watch on television. Then came the long night again.

I also received visits from three others. One was my colleague, Steven Kenyon, from Birkdale School. He lived in Matlock so it was not too far to come and see me. He, no doubt, kept colleagues at Birkdale informed. In fact, Sarah and I received regular telephone calls from my Headmaster, Robert Court, at Birkdale.

Another former colleague, from Mill Hill School, Tony Rosser, came to see me in hospital and at home. I will always be grateful for him taking the time to see me when at that time he had duties as Mayor of Matlock.

Finally, my friend from school, John, came to see me when I was having my second course of IVE chemotherapy in January 2004. All of their support greatly helped to keep my spirits up.

During this stay in hospital I had a lot of time to think, particularly as I was in a room on my own. On one occasion I was listening to BBC Radio 2 through my Walkman. It was the Jeremy Vine show which I enjoyed for the informative debates. One of the records played was *Reflections of My Life* by *The Marmalade*. This is a sad song which made me reflect on what had happened to me. It also contains the lines:

All my sorrow, sad tomorrows, take me back to my own home.

All my crying, feel I'm dying, take me back to my own home.

It also says in another line:

I'm changing, I'm changing everything around me.

These words seemed to sum up my feelings at this point that my life was never going to be the same again and I was mourning for the life which seemed to be lost.

The final day of chemotherapy was on 29 November which was my 43rd birthday. I seemed fated to be at a hospital on my birthday as had been the case in 1995.

Sarah had left my presents the day before so that I could open them on my birthday. However on the morning of my birthday I felt a little nauseous and spaced out, and for the first time my appetite was reduced. I felt miserable that I was still in hospital for my birthday. However, the day got better.

At least I was expected to be able to go home in the afternoon when the final bag of chemotherapy had been completed. This cheered me up. Also, in the morning, the hospital had a jam sponge birthday cake sent up for me from the kitchen. I then received a surprise telephone call from a former teaching colleague at my previous school, Mill Hill. News had spread about my relapse from Tony and two more former colleagues wanted to visit me before I went home.

I was glad to be coming home. However, on the way home Sarah dropped in a letter to our GP, Dr Skidmore. In the car I had my birthday cake on my lap. For a split second at a traffic queue Sarah glanced down at the cake. As she set off a car in front stopped suddenly and Sarah almost drove into the back of it. I shouted, 'Look out!'. Sarah said, 'Thank goodness you are not as spaced out as I thought you were'.

When I finally arrived at home I then had another visit, this time from Julie, a colleague from Birkdale School who brought me a birthday card and a box of Cadbury's Heroes for us all to share. She had interrupted her weekend break at Center Park to see me. In the end, a day I had dreaded turned out to be quite a pleasant birthday. It made us all feel the happiest we had felt for weeks. However, Sarah wanted to cook me something special but all I could fancy were a few salmon sandwiches. However I did manage to drink a slither of wine!

In the next few days I felt tired but happy that the first cycle of chemotherapy was completed and that my kidneys were now functioning normally. By Tuesday 2 December I felt quite well and even cooked a meal for Sarah. On Wednesday I started to shiver, though I did not think anything of it.

By the Thursday my temperature was rising which signalled my greatest fear; it appeared that I had developed an infection. Chemotherapy makes your blood counts fall dramatically - I would be neutraphenic suggesting that my white blood counts and neutraphils were very low. As these are necessary to fight bacterial infections I was open to any infection.

By the evening I felt hot and cold and my temperature went above 38°C. The doctors at the hospital had told me that this was the point when I needed to be admitted to hospital.

Sarah had gone to college and I had to telephone her on the mobile. She immediately came back and I telephoned Ward 10 at the Derbyshire Royal Infirmary who told me to come in. Sarah told me later on that at about 8.15 that evening she had a feeling that something was wrong. This was about the time my temperature reached the dreaded level and I made the decision to contact Ward 10. This psychic perception was to occur again when I was having my stem cell transplant.

Luckily our friend Nina who offered to come and sit with me whilst Sarah was at college was able to stay and look after Dominic. Sarah then took me to Derby at 10.00 p.m. I was blood tested and examined by a junior doctor on call and a bed was found. I was then put on antibiotic drips for the next few days. Sarah told me afterwards that when she left me at about 11.30 p.m. the entrance to the hospital was blocked by a number of cars. Sarah thought they might be drug dealers. This was very frightening for her. Eventually they dispersed and she was able to get out.

On the Friday I felt very ill. My temperature shot up to 38.8°C and I just lay curled up on the bed. It had proved to be the right decision to inform the hospital; an infection could have been very dangerous for me because my immune system was suppressed.

It then turned out that Sarah could not come and see me for a few days as she had developed a sore throat and cold which could have been dangerous to me with a zero white blood count and very low neutraphils. It made me feel very low.

My spirits were further reduced when my Hickman Line fell out on the Monday. I was washing my hands after going to the toilet when I noticed the white tube hanging down. It was a complete shock to me but apparently this can happen if the skin has not grown properly around the line. I had only just had the second set of stitches removed which made it vulnerable. This made me feel very miserable because I knew that it would mean a longer stay in Ward 10 since a new Hickman Line would have to be fitted. I had been hoping to be well enough to come out and see Dominic's nativity play at school but it was not to be.

To add to this the doctors told me I was to have a bone marrow biopsy to assess what progress had been made after the first cycle of chemotherapy. I had always dreaded this but I was told further that I could not have a sedative as I had had for the previous biopsies. This was because somewhere in the country a patient had suffered an adverse reaction, so sedatives were now banned for bone marrow biopsies.

I therefore realised that I was going to experience some pain although Addy, the Registrar who conducted the biopsy, was very gentle and kept apologising when he thought that his actions were causing me pain.

On the Thursday I had my second Hickman Line fitted. Unfortunately it was not as straightforward as the first time. There was a great deal of bleeding afterwards from my neck. In the afternoon I had a visit from Roy, a Baptist minster from Swanwick. I suddenly began bleeding again as he arrived. He had to run into the corridor to fetch a nurse because I could not reach the buzzer with blood oozing all over my chest. I was very grateful to Roy because this was the second time he had come to see me in hospital. Each time he offered me a prayer which seemed to offer comfort.

Friday 12 December was a very low day for me. It started badly when I discovered masses of hair on the pillow so I knew that my hair was starting to fall out. This is always a bad point with chemotherapy. You expect it to happen but it seems such a blow when it does.

Then came a bombshell; the doctors came on the rounds and told me that I needed to come into hospital on Christmas Eve to begin the second cycle of IVE chemotherapy. There should not be more than a four-week gap between cycles otherwise the good work of the previous one might be undone. I needed to be admitted on Christmas Eve to begin the second course so that the cycle would be right to collect stem cells in early January at Nottingham City Hospital; apparently, the stem cells needed to be collected one week after the course of chemotherapy had ended and then frozen. Since the laboratory at Nottingham was closed at certain times over the Christmas period the window for collecting them was only a short one.

I had been led to believe two days earlier that my next treatment was to begin on New Year's Eve. Christmas Eve was unacceptable with a six-year-old child. Santa cannot be in hospital! When you have a six-year-old you value Christmas because you cannot be sure when he will stop believing in Santa and then the magic of Christmas will fade. When I told Sarah she was very angry and stormed out of the room. She told me afterwards she needed some space and did not want to vent her anger on me.

My mother and father also arrived with Sarah and tried to comfort her. I was then visited by Alan, who stressed the importance of not delaying the next treatment. The air was filled with tension. Dr Maine tried to relieve this by cracking a joke about sending me a bill for the new Hickman Line! The doctors thought the disease was now more aggressive and I might not be here next Christmas if I did not take it seriously. It must have been awful for my parents to have been present when I was informed of this. My mother seemed to have been much stronger this time and in 2001; more than I had expected. However I was later told that when they went home with Sarah there was a flow of tears from my mother. My father kept his feelings more bottled up but on many occasions when he visited me in hospital I could see him looking at me and I suspect he was thinking, 'Why are you in hospital when I am 75 years old and you are only 43 years old?'.

My mother would also say on many occasions, 'I wish I could take this illness from you'. It must be part of a parent's love because I used to say on many occasions, 'I would rather it be me suffering with this illness than Dominic'.

As might be imagined, this was a real low point and it presented me with a terrible dilemma. I could take a chance on the illness returning if I left the second cycle another week. If that occurred I would miss the slot for my stem cell harvest which was crucial to the long-term treatment. On the other hand, everything might be fine and I need not spend time in hospital at Christmas.

The misery continued; I was informed that lunch was cancelled because I was to have a CT scan in the afternoon. I felt very miserable sitting in the waiting area for the scan, particularly as I was next to a Christmas tree. I felt like smashing it down and forgetting all about Christmas. Christmas is a hard time to be ill. I was, and still am, not a great fan of Christmas but when I was in hospital and observed decorations and Christmas trees in every corridor and on the ward I could not bear to look at them.

At least there was some good news. After the CT scan, and once my dressing had been checked, I could go home that day. My temperature was now normal and blood counts recovering.

This stay in hospital was by far my worst. I felt shell-shocked afterwards. It left me feeling very low, and uncertain of the future. For the first time, I wondered whether I might actually die from this illness. It took a few days to recover but as time went by I rediscovered my positive attitude. I was going to win through in the end.

We discussed how we might salvage Christmas and agreed to tell Dominic that Santa sometimes has to come a day earlier to certain boys and girls. We also agreed to have Christmas dinner on Christmas Eve.

On Wednesday 17 December I attended the Day Case Unit at Derby to have my bloods checked. I was able to drive myself which was encouraging. There was good news in that my blood counts were recovering nicely. Furthermore, the CT scan had revealed a good reduction in the size of the stomach lymph nodes and the bone marrow was improved. Then came even better news; Dr McKernan had consulted with Dr Haynes at Nottingham City Hospital and it was agreed that my next cycle of chemotherapy could be left until New Year's Eve. I was prescribed some steroids which was like a mini dose of chemotherapy to keep the disease at bay.

Imagine how our spirits soared! To celebrate we had a lovely Christmas meal at lunchtime on the Thursday. Sarah said that it was nice to do something normal for a change. It meant a lot to her that I had made the effort.

Sarah and I were now determined to have a good Christmas. It was the first piece of good news in weeks. It made our Christmas, knowing that progress had been made against the disease once again. Although my red blood count was still on the low side I seemed to gather strength. I felt tired around Christmas Eve and on Christmas Day but I had always found Christmas Day tiring at the best of times. However, from Boxing Day until I went back to Ward 10 I picked up. I felt much better, in fact, the best I had felt for months. I was able to find strength to play with Dominic and his toys. We had a wonderful two weeks when I was not in hospital and could have a normal family life. It is amazing what we take for granted. Normal family life is much more appreciated after periods of illness and disruption.

We received a further bonus on New Year's Eve. The hospital telephoned to say that the chemotherapy would not be ready for another day so I did not need to be admitted until the evening of New Year's Day. Sarah's face lit up.

We spent a pleasant New Year's Evening and Day together. When I went in for my second cycle of IVE chemotherapy I was in much better spirits and Sarah felt able to take me this time. Consequently, I seemed to sail though the five days. There were few problems except for some blood in the urine.

This better period seemed to continue when I came out of hospital on 6 January 2004. This time I was given preventative antibiotics, antiviral and antifungal tablets to prevent me developing a temperature and having to be admitted again. The hospital were concerned that I should be able to produce my stem cell harvest on time which was to be one week after the end of this cycle of chemotherapy. The scene of the action was then about to switch to Nottingham City Hospital.

CHAPTER 10
Stem Cells and Frustrations

After my return home on 6 January the cocktail of tablets I was given seemed to keep me well following the second cycle of IVE chemotherapy. I assumed that the doctors needed me to stay well so that they could mobilise the stem cell harvest. On Friday 9 January I was blood tested at Derby and discovered that I was already neutraphenic. I therefore held my breath over the weekend and hoped for no bacterial infection. My temperature did rise to 37.5°C on the Sunday evening but then returned to normal. It was so important that I should able to attend Nottingham City Hospital on the Monday morning.

I was to attend every day at Nottingham until stem cells had been harvested and frozen. The body's bone marrow is suppressed during chemotherapy, hence the low blood counts. However once it begins to recover, new 'baby' or 'command' cells are produced which are stem cells. They can move in the body to wherever they are needed to repair damaged organs. There is much discussion about the use of embryonic stem cells to restore body organs and cure diseases. However, there are ethical arguments about using unborn foetuses. In my case, as the stem cells were generated from adult bone marrow no such ethical issues arose.

The stem cells were to be collected and frozen; they would then be used at a later date when I was given high-dose chemotherapy. This would just about destroy the bone marrow which would normally take months to repair itself. At this stage, the stem cells would be dripped back into the body and would act as seeds to regenerate the bone marrow. So, the successful harvesting of my stem cells was critical.

I needed hospital transport to make the journey to Nottingham City Hospital Haematology Day Case Unit. I felt too weak after the second cycle of chemotherapy to drive and Sarah could not take me because of getting Dominic to school.

It was not expected that stem cells would be harvested on day one. However I was blood tested and was horrified when informed that my red blood count was only 7.4 (normal range 11.5-15). My white blood count was only 0.12 and platelets only 6. They should have been at least 150; at such a low level, any cut would have had great difficulty in clotting.

I was informed that I would be sent off to Derby in the afternoon to receive some blood and platelets urgently. Before setting off I was shown the stem cell room and the machine which would extract them. It simply looked like a large washing machine with many tubes. I was also warned that I would need to consume some milky products before going on the machine because it depleted calcium levels and could cause tingling in the body. If this did occur they could provide me with calcium tablets.

After this I was sent off in a taxi to Derby. I did warn the driver to drive steadily because if the car crashed I would probably bleed to death. I do not think she quite believed me! Thankfully, I stayed calm during the journey.

I arrived safely at Derby and was given the blood and platelets. Whilst I was there, a lady came in with family or friends. She very obviously had an extremely heavy cold. I was filled with fear because with such a low white blood count I was very vulnerable. I discreetly informed the nursing staff who whisked her and her family off to a cubicle. I felt bad about acting so selfishly but I knew what the consequences might have been had I picked up this virus; another stay in hospital at the very least. I do not know whether this lady was a patient herself or a relative of a patient but either way, in her condition she should not have been allowed to come near patients who might have been receiving chemotherapy and who would therefore be highly vulnerable to infection.

There were no more scares and Sarah came and picked me up at the end of the afternoon. On the Tuesday my white blood count was still only 0.25 and there were no stem cells so I was sent home.

By Wednesday the white blood count was only 0.47 and still no stem cells so again I was sent home. At this point Dr Haynes suggested that I doubled the GCSF injections. These were to boost the bone marrow into producing more white blood cells. I needed a white blood count of at least 1.0 before they could extract any stem cells.

This seemed to do the trick because on the Thursday my white blood count had jumped to 2.2 and stem cells were detected at last. In the afternoon I was put on the stem cell machine for the first time. I had a tube attached to each of the valves on my Hickman Line. One of these took blood out of my body and fed it into the machine which extracted the stem cells. It then returned the blood minus the stem cells through the other tube. The whole process took about three and a half hours and at the end of the afternoon I was informed that about four million stem cells had been harvested. The nursing staff were very pleased because they had estimated that it was likely only to be one million. On the Friday another eight million stem cells were harvested and then I was given blood in the afternoon because my red blood count was still only 8.4.

By the end of the week I was very pleased with the results but I was also very tired. In the following week Sarah and I finally met Dr Andy Haynes at the clinic at Nottingham on 21 January. He was and still is a very impressive Consultant and gave us a biology lesson in how my illness had transformed itself into Non-Hodgkin's Lymphoma T-cell enriched B. We did not know what it meant but understood it was more serious. We were to discover that he did not pull punches. He came straight to the point.

We were given a prognosis; without the final high-dose chemotherapy and stem cell transplant there would only be a 15% chance of the illness *not* returning and, therefore, an 85% chance that it *would* return in a few months. With the stem cell transplant there was a 65% chance of complete cure or five years in remission although if the disease did return it would be more difficult to treat because the number of cells would be greater. If a transplant went ahead the medical team had decided to use my own stem cells rather than those from a donor as this involved less risk in terms of mortality from infections. However, to use a donor's stem cells would reduce the risk of the illness coming back even further. We agreed with the decision to use my own stem cells because the mortality rate was then only 1%. Also my stem cells would be screened and hence should be cancer-free when they were put in.

The odds were reasonable, although not as good as we might have hoped for. Sarah was very quiet. She told me afterwards that the 1% mortality rate worried her but there seemed to be no alternative. She knew my teaching days were definitely over. The prognosis confirmed my decision to seek medical retirement from teaching. Dr Haynes was a firm believer in the link between stress and a reduction in the immune system which reduced the ability of the body's natural defence system to fight cancer. I also thought that if there was a possibility that the disease might return and be more difficult to treat then I may as well enjoy life rather than return to the pressures of full-time work for no real gain. I therefore submitted my retirement forms that week. I was concerned that my age would be against me but, after hearing Dr Haynes, I believed that the hospital report should make out a convincing case in my favour.

After seeing Dr Haynes, a frustrating waiting game began which was to last for weeks. We were surprised to learn from Dr Haynes that he would not sanction the stem cell transplant unless there had been at least a 50% reduction in the stomach lymph nodes and until the bone marrow was clear or there was little involvement. I was therefore to have more scans.

During these weeks my Hickman Line had to be maintained. It needed to be flushed each week to ensure that there was no clotting. There was also a dressing to be changed to prevent infection entering the opening where the tube went into my chest. Thankfully I had a wonderful district nurse called Anita who was very confident in dealing with this. She was also a cheerful positive influence whenever she entered the house.

There was also a great fear of the Hickman Line falling out again. I needed it for my stem cell transplant and it became an obsession to look at it every day to check it was alright. One night I had a dream that I was pulling it out and woke up in a sweat to rush to the bathroom mirror to check that it was still there!

On 28 January I had another painful bone marrow biopsy at Derby. However, the sample in the jar looked good. On 4 February I had a CT scan, also at Derby. I then had to wait until 16 February to see Dr Haynes at Nottingham again. It was a return to waiting for things to happen and the resumption of frustrations.

Firstly, obtaining the biopsy results proved not to be straightforward. I had to telephone Derby on a number of occasions. On Friday 6 February Alan was able to tell me that the bone marrow was clear which was excellent news. However, the full CT scan was not available. Alan thought that the stomach lymph nodes were okay but there was something else in the groin that had shown up on the scan. They were unsure whether it was lymphatic fluid from my operations or a new lump. He said I should not worry and that he was booking me in for Dr Haynes anyway. This did plant seeds of doubt in my mind, however. I started to worry that there might be further delays and that the illness might start creeping back.

At the same time I discovered that my application for retirement on medical grounds had broken down. The forms had been returned to school and I was told that another set needed to be filled in. I then telephoned Dr McKernan's secretary at Derby to let her know that this different form was on its way only to discover that the hospital report had not been started. This was a relief in a way because it avoided the embarrassment of asking Dr McKernan to complete fresh forms but it was also frustrating because I so desperately wanted to sort out medical retirement before Easter otherwise there would be financial problems in the summer.

I felt very deflated because everything seemed to be going wrong. It seemed to be a time when every event of great importance in my life was completely out of my control. However, just as quickly, things started to happen. The report was passed to Dr Maine and he completed it very promptly. The Bursar at Birkdale School and Dr Maine's secretary at Derby then cut through the red tape and made the Teacher's Pension Organisation realise that someone facing a stem cell transplant should not have to be going though this agony of indecision and frustration. On 19 February medical retirement was granted. It was a day of mixed feelings. I had not wanted my teaching career to end like this but it was a relief that I would not have to go back to the pressures of the job and risk the illness returning again.

The appointment to see Dr Haynes at clinic again finally came round. There was a long wait before we discovered that no scan results had been sent from Derby. I then had to wait another hour.

Dr Haynes only had the CT scan results but he spotted the concern about the groin. He checked the area and thought that there might be a small lump. However, he was happy enough with my progress to book me into the system for the transplant. He thought that this might take place in the following week.

Once the medical retirement was granted and other problems were sorted out my mind was clear. The doctors at Derby wanted to ultrasound the groin to determine exactly what the situation was. However no date was available until 25 February. In the event the ultrasound scan never took place. On Monday 23rd Dr Haynes telephoned me to let me know that I would be admitted to Fletcher Ward at Nottingham City Hospital at some point that week. He was unconcerned about the ultrasound examination and stated that it would not stop the transplant going ahead.

On the morning of Thursday 26 February I was admitted to Fletcher Ward. I knew the process was going to be difficult; I had been warned by Dr Haynes of horrendous side-effects. I was also expected to be in hospital for three weeks. However, I wanted to get on with it and get the job completed so that we could all return to a normal life.

CHAPTER 11
The Final Battle

On Thursday 26 February 2004 I was admitted to Fletcher Ward in Nottingham City Hospital. Upon arrival I was greeted by Dan, a male nurse, and shown to my room. It was a modern, pleasant ward with a widescreen television, hi-fi system and an electronic adjustable bed. There were only two beds in the room meaning it would be quiet, but with someone there to talk to. Sarah stayed with me until lunch time. She was very calm in front of me as we met Sutchi, my Registrar, who explained what would happen. She made us both feel very calm about what was to happen because we both knew it was going to be an ordeal. However, Sarah told me after I came out of hospital that she had tears in her eyes as soon as she left the building until reaching the car. It could not have been easy for her knowing that I could be in Fletcher Ward for up to three weeks.

On the first day blood tests were carried out and then after lunch I was taken for a heart scan. This was deemed necessary because of the strain the high-dose chemotherapy would place on my heart. This time the regime would consist of four drugs: Cytarabine, Carmustine, Etoposide and Melphalan. These drugs would eradicate any remaining cancer cells but were so powerful that they would greatly reduce the bone marrow function. The stem cells were to be administered immediately after completion as 'seeds' to regenerate the bone marrow. Without these stem cells the bone marrow would take many months to recover.

Each of these drugs had the usual side-effects of lowered blood counts, nausea, vomiting and hair loss. There was also the additional hazard of diarrhoea which was not a problem I had encountered with previous chemotherapy regimes.

In the late afternoon I was given the first bag of chemotherapy, Carmustine, to be administered intravenously through the Hickman Line. This lasted two hours. It made me feel a little strange during the process but I felt fine after it stopped.

I was also started on a cocktail of tablets and syrups to protect me against bacterial and viral infections because, as with all chemotherapies I had received so far, my immune system would become vulnerable. Over the weeks in the ward I grew to hate taking these. Four times a day these syrups and tablets would arrive at my table; morning, noon, teatime and evening. The syrups tasted revolting and some of the tablets were so large that I dreaded choking on them. I found myself breaking some of the tablets in half so that I could swallow them.

Often I would lie in my bed and look at the tablets before I could drum up the courage to attempt to take them. Sometimes the temptation was there to flush them away down a toilet but I was afraid that if I did not take them there would be serious consequences. I also needed many glasses of water to help swallow the tablets and swill the taste of the syrups away. It felt as though I needed gallons of water. Swallowing tablets became a particular problem when my throat and mouth became sore as my white blood count declined. My biggest fear was that I would vomit them up and then the necessary drugs would not be entering my blood stream, protecting me as they should.

On days two, three, four and five of my stay in Fletcher Ward there was a pattern of chemotherapy of a two-hour bag dripped in during the middle of the day between 11.30 am and 1.30 pm. This was the Etoposide drug. Later on, at 10.00 p.m., I received the drug Cytarabine which took about 20 minutes to drip in.

Day six was when the potentially most potent drug, Melphalan, was administered. Although it took only five minutes to administer through the Hickman Line I was made to suck ice lollies for about one hour beforehand and for about half an hour afterwards. This was because this particular chemotherapy could cause bad ulcers in the mouth and throat and ice constricts the blood vessels, preventing this. As a child I had never been a great fan of ice lollies and after this I felt I would never want another for the remainder of my life! Julie was my nurse that day and I remember her telling me off, not for failing to take medicine, but for not eating enough ice lollies!

This completed the programme of high-dose chemotherapy. Twenty-four hours later at about 12.30 p.m. on Wednesday 3 March I was given my stem cell transplant, administered intravenously through the Hickman Line. This was a poignant moment because these were the seeds which would regenerate the bone marrow once the chemotherapy had suppressed it. It is a painless process but one which apparently leaves you smelling of sweetcorn for a few days although at the time I could not smell it myself - but it might explain the lack of visitors for a few days! For some reason Sarah could not smell it either. A few days later the patient I was sharing with, Bob, had his stem cells administered and I could smell him for days, and this was at a time when I felt sickly, the effects of the chemotherapy having kicked in. Apparently the smell comes from the substance in which the stem cells are stored. When they were administered the bag looked as if it was full of tomato sauce.

After my stem cells were administered it was then a matter of waiting for my blood counts to fall and my immune system to depress. It is an awful feeling knowing that you are going to become ill but not knowing what form the symptoms will take.

Up to then I had felt reasonably well but there had been two early problems. From Monday 1 March I started to suffer from diarrhoea which became severe after a few days. The nurses gave me some tablets initially but later dripped in something stronger because of its severity. However, it never really abated for 12 days until I went home.

The second problem was the emergence of spots all over my legs, arms and chest. The Registrar diagnosed folliculitis. This is a bacterial infection of the hair follicles in the body where hair had dropped out from previous chemotherapy treatments. Unfortunately, you do not lose just the hair on your head but body hairs all over, leaving the follicles vulnerable to infections. The spots did not itch but looked unsightly so I was given some antibiotics to remove the problem. Unfortunately, these probably added to the effects of the chemotherapy to worsen the diarrhoea

Despite these problems I felt fine and was eating very well. The food was good and plentiful and with little physical activity I put on weight in the first week and a half I was on Fletcher Ward. I saw my Consultant, Dr Haynes, on Friday 5th and he stated that I should expect to feel ill by Monday. If I did not, the treatment was not working!

True enough I noticed a change on the Sunday when my appetite started to decline and I felt more tired. My brother Martin and his wife Debbie came to see me and I began to feel that I could not cope with visitors as tiredness crept in.

The diarrhoea was also bad despite the drips and I started to feel some nausea. Nowadays there are very good anti-sickness drugs and I suspect the problem is not as bad as it was for patients in the past. However, with such a high dose of chemotherapy it was perhaps inevitable that I would have some feelings of sickness.

By the Monday, as forecast, I did feel very ill. Sarah came to see me and I think that she was shocked. I could hardly lift my head off the pillow and felt very sleepy. Even so, every morning I forced myself to have a bath because of the diarrhoea. It was important to feel clean.

Sarah found it very hard to see me like this. She was very worried because she remembered that there was a 1% mortality risk. However, she knew that I was a fighter!

It was also difficult that morning to feel cheerful about anything. At about 8.00 a.m. before Sarah came, she put Dominic on the telephone to talk to me. He was bursting to tell me that he had lost his first baby tooth and the tooth fairy had given him *50p*! I found it very difficult to be cheerful with him. I did not want him to realise that his daddy felt so poorly. It was good that members of my family could telephone me directly because I had a telephone with an extension next to my bed. However, I did not always want to talk to them when I felt ill. My brother Mike telephoned me at about 4.30 p.m. that day. I had woken up from a sleep and felt dreadful. He must have been quite shocked that I sounded so weary and rushed him off the telephone. I felt bad about this afterwards because it must have been hard for my family in Hull when they could not see me. Unfortunately, that week my father was also admitted to hospital in Hull with serious skin problems. This was the start of a four-week stay in hospital for him. This was an additional worry but I knew there was nothing I could do. As a result, no-one could come down to see me that week from Hull. Poor Sarah had to bear all of the suffering I was enduring. I was thankful for a visit on the Tuesday from my former colleague, Tony, and my long-time school friend, John, on the Saturday. John once again came up from Leicester to see me. I will always appreciate those who put themselves out to visit me. I also appreciate those who gave Sarah support in any way. Not everyone did. Sarah and I sometimes felt that some people could not face cancer and seeing me. You realise when you are ill who really cares about you.

My temperature was also rising suggesting an infection. This helped to make me feel sleepy. This was expected as my immune system became depressed as the bone marrow was suppressed. My white blood count and neutraphils were falling and were close to zero by Monday and were completely flat on Tuesday. Whilst in the ward, temperature and blood pressure readings were taken at regular intervals every day from day one. This would start at 6.15 in the morning! My blood was also tested regularly with a nurse wanting a blood sample also at 6.15 a.m.! I was at least offered a cup of tea as a peace offering.

When the immune system was depressed it had implications for visitors. People were not supposed to come near if they had any sign of a cold or other infection. If they did, they had to wear a mask which was provided by the hospital. Also, everyone had to bathe their hands in an alcohol-based agent as they came onto the ward and as they left, again to prevent any risk of infections to patients. One effect of this was that I never saw Dominic from Tuesday 1 March until Saturday 13 March because he had a cough. I missed him terribly but then I did not feel like a six-year-old crawling all over me. Another effect was that when Sarah came she had to wear a mask, as did Dominic when he finally came to see me.

Monday 8 March was the start of a period of four days when I felt very ill. I would describe this period as the worst four days of my life so far. My day consisted of getting up and having a bath. Sarah would then visit me in the morning and in the afternoon I would watch television. Often I would sleep. Sometimes, while asleep on top of the bed some diarrhoea would creep out and when I awoke my pyjama bottoms would feel damp. I would realise then what had happened and that it had soiled the bedclothes. On one occasion when this happened I had the embarrassment of attempting to get to the toilet to clean myself up. I had to walk past the bed of the patient who shared the room and he had a number of visitors around his bed. I hoped that they would not notice my wet pyjama bottoms as I walked past!

This was very embarrassing and degrading. However, when I called the nurses they were very understanding and told me that it was very common and not to worry. In fact the nurses were all marvellous on Fletcher Ward. I believe that most nurses in the NHS are very dedicated and deserve much greater reward than they actually receive. I was totally dependent on them and they were magnificent.

The diarrhoea was perhaps the worst part of this treatment for me. In addition to the little accidents I would have to get up several times in the night and when I had a temperature it made me feel very weak. I felt that I was dying and on several occasions in the middle of the night wished that I had not started this treatment. I felt that I would never be well again but I had to dig deep in my reserves of determination. I had no choice but to battle and go forward and eventually, things did improve.

On Monday and Tuesday during the night I felt hot with the high temperature. I drifted in and out of sleep. During the early hours of Tuesday morning I imagined that there were people moving about under the bed. When you are delirious your mind plays tricks.

On the Wednesday I did feel a little better although my appetite was still flat. There was a glimmer of hope in that I was informed that my white blood count and neutraphils were starting to turn. It was forecast that by Saturday I should start to feel better; the stem cell seeds were starting to germinate!

However the diarrhoea continued and my temperature was still high at 39°C. It was then suggested by the Registrar that there might be a fungal infection so I was to be given an antifungal drip. I was also warned that this could cause an allergic reaction and if I experienced any feelings of shivering, the nursing staff needed to be called immediately. On the Thursday I would find out why.

That next day I actually felt a little better again but I was still not eating and the diarrhoea was still a problem although it was beginning to ease even though the motions had changed colour to green. Perhaps this was because of the antifungal drug.

That evening I was given a stronger dose of the antifungal drug. Everything seemed fine until about three hours into the drip (which took four hours in all to administer). I developed the allergic reaction. I had been to the toilet at about 7.30 and settled down on my bed to watch television. Suddenly I began to shiver and so, as instructed, I called the nurses. The shivering became very violent, unlike anything I had ever experienced before. Dan and Julie, the two nurses just starting night duty, reacted immediately. Dan quickly prepared antihistamine and hydrocortisone injections which were administered into the Hickman Line. Julie covered me in blankets and I was given oxygen because my breathing became too fast and the level of oxygen in the blood was falling too low. Eventually, after about 15 minutes - although to me it seemed much longer - the shaking settled down and then I felt very hot for the remainder of the evening. Apparently, the allergic reaction had spiked my temperature up suddenly. That was certainly a scary experience. I later asked if it could have killed me without the injections. There was no answer.

On the Friday I felt better and my temperature was settling down. I also managed to eat a small amount of food, the first time since Sunday that I had eaten. The worst appeared to be over. Sarah came to see me in the afternoon. She told me that at college the previous evening she had experienced a feeling of panic at about the time I was experiencing the reaction. It makes you believe that you have found your soul mate when this sort of thing occurs. This was the second time she had been at college and sensed that I was feeling ill; the previous occasion had been in December.

That Friday afternoon I was given an unexpected boost. Dr Haynes came to see me on his rounds and informed me that my white blood count and neutraphils were rising and that there was a possibility that I could go home over the weekend. After the dramatic week I had experienced this would have seemed extremely unlikely 24 hours earlier. The stem cell seeds had obviously taken and the bone marrow was recovering.

However my red blood and platelet counts were still low. I was given two bags of blood and platelets on the Thursday and Friday. It had been expected that I would need these at some point. The red blood and platelet counts seemed to decline after the white blood count and neutraphils. For some reason the red blood cells seem to decline more slowly.

I was given a further boost when my friend John once again came up from Leicester to see me. By then I was feeling more sociable and able to see visitors.

On Sunday 14 March I was allowed home by the duty Registrar. It was such a relief after such a long stretch in hospital. My mother and brother Mike picked me up. It was a pleasure to step out and see the spring sunshine again although I felt very weak. I was warned that there would be at least a three-month recovery period and it would be six months before my immune system would be as it should.

The first week at home was difficult with poor appetite, poor sleep, some feelings of nausea and the sheer feeling of weakness. I found it difficult to settle and Sarah was fearful of the huge responsibility that lay upon her shoulders. However, at least the treatment was over; I was so pleased to be back with Sarah and Dominic and that the period of recovery could begin.

This progressed well through April and May although my red blood count remained on the low side. In May I felt well enough to make two visits to Birkdale School, the first since October 2003. I wanted to see my colleagues again and explain to my pupils why they had been without my services for so long. Everyone was delighted to see me. It felt like I had conquered adversity and it was a triumphant return after a war. However I was no longer a teacher there after my medical retirement began on 26 April.

The diarrhoea problem improved initially. However, I was put on two preventative antibiotics for at least three months, and for one course it was four months and by June and July this had made my bowels bad again with some diarrhoea. The antibiotics also made me feel tired with a variable appetite.

On 12 July Sarah and I were invited as guests to Birkdale School Speech Day. I wanted to go to this event but had visions of running out of the hall to the toilet during the Headmaster's speech. Thankfully, this did not occur!

On 16 July I returned to Birkdale School on the last day of term to join my colleagues for an end-of-term lunch. I was also to receive some leaving gifts and needed to make a speech. Sarah thought that this would be difficult for me as not only was I leaving Birkdale, I was also leaving teaching as a career.

In the event, the speech flowed quite easily. I realised that I had really left many months earlier. It was not as though I had been teaching up to that day. It was also the day that I had dreamed about when I was in my hospital bed on Fletcher Ward. It was a day that I had looked forward to as an opportunity to explain to everyone what had happened. It was also a day I had dreaded because this was the final curtain on my career.

It came as a shock to discover at a check-up clinic on 19 July that my white blood count and neutraphils were quite low again. It was explained to me by the Registrar that these effects were due to the antibiotics and were not unexpected. In fact, in the week before I attended clinic I had experienced a rash around the neck. Luckily I was almost at the end of the course of antibiotics.

As part of the recovery I was scanned to assess how successful the treatment had been. I was given a dreaded bone marrow biopsy in May and was told on 24 May that this was clear. In fact, at that point Dr Haynes was very pleased with my progress. On 1 June I had a CT scan; I was given the results on 21 June and was told that the stomach and groin lymph nodes were clear of cancer. I was in remission again, although Dr Haynes simply said that the disease was 'under control'. I was told to get on with my life once more. However, life was never to be the same again.

CHAPTER 12
Looking Back, Looking Forward

The third relapse of Lymphoma left a significant legacy. It was to bring about a huge change in my life. Firstly I had retired from teaching on medical grounds because Sarah and I were convinced of the link between stress and the development of Non-Hodgkin's Lymphoma. No one can say for certain what causes a cancer but each time my Lymphoma developed, it followed periods of considerable pressure and stress, even though I had not realised that I was suffering in this way at the time.

Another aspect is the shadow such illness casts. After the first onset I did not expect that it would come back again. After the second, I had felt so well, and had been given a drug which seemed to be so effective, that I believed it would not return although I could not be totally sure. After this third time, I want to believe that it has gone forever but there is always a part of the mind where there is doubt. I do think about whether it might come back. I also worry about whether other cancers might develop. I was warned before all of my chemotherapy treatments that they in themselves could cause other cancers. However, what choice did I have?

The time around the approach of a routine clinic appointment is always tense. Any changes in my health start to plant seeds of concern. Sarah in particular gets stressed if I have any illness which will not clear up quickly.

Dr Haynes stated on one of my regular clinic visits that things have changed and that I should enjoy life. I took this as a warning but I am an optimist now that a great source of stress is removed from my life. Time will tell if medically retiring from teaching was the correct decision.

I also felt for a few months that I could not go through the treatment again in the future. The stem cell transplant in particular made me feel very ill and I said to everyone immediately afterwards that I could not go through such a treatment again. However, when you have your family to live for I suppose you would go through it again if you had to. I do know that another relapse would mean a donor's stem cells or bone marrow. This would bring the new worry of finding a donor - I already know that neither of my two brothers is a match.

As I look back on the whole experience I feel that my whole outlook on life has changed. One positive change has been the influence of those with whom I have been brought into contact. I have met so many poorly people, many worse than myself. Most of them have been so brave, positive and cheerful they are an inspiration. Although I wish that I had never encountered this dreadful illness I feel that it has been a privilege to meet such people. I felt I was privileged to be suffering with them. This has inspired me to seek voluntary work offering support to newly-diagnosed lymphoma patients through the Lymphoma Association. They are, of course, one of the beneficiaries of the profits from this book.

Another positive outcome is my appreciation for those in the world who do good work. It is easy to turn on the news every day and see violence and confrontation and be tempted into into thinking that the whole world is rotten. I have seen so much good work going on by all doctors and nurses in the Derby and Nottingham hospitals where I have been treated that I now feel that the world has a great number of good people. This is further reinforced when I think about the transfusions of red blood and platelets that I have received. I will never know who donated the blood. People who donate blood and bone marrow are indeed wonderful and I am eternally grateful to whoever my donors were. I suppose you could say that my faith in humanity has been restored by meeting fellow patients and health workers.

Another positive outcome is that Sarah and I are not motivated so much by money these days. After developing a cancer you realise that it does not matter how much money you have in the bank. It will not buy you good health. Cancer also does not discriminate according to financial circumstances. When I medically retired it involved a drop in income but this does not matter as long as we can survive. I am lucky in that I have a good teaching pension. Many fellow cancer sufferers I have spoken to have experienced financial worries in addition to the uncertainties of their illness. I was fortunate. My life has became much easier and I can now do the things I want to do without waiting until I am too old to do them, albeit within tighter financial constraints.

Sarah and I both now feel that it is important to do something useful and worthwhile with the time gained by my retirement. I have sought voluntary work as by helping others I feel I can do some good. In September 2005 I became secretary for a haematology patient support group at Nottingham City Hospital. We called our group H.O.P.E. which stands for Haematology Open Patient Enquiries. The group is made up of patients like myself and some hospital staff. We all aim to help patients who are diagnosed with any blood disorders because a Haematology Department does not only treat blood cancers. The group is ultimately aiming to provide support for patients on clinic days and to provide 'buddying' support for patients who need a longer chat. We feel we can all make a difference because we have 'been there'.

Becoming secretary for this group has made me feel important and useful again. Medically retiring at the age of forty-three left a 'hole' in my life. I was glad to be alive and well again but I needed to have a purpose in life. H.O.P.E. has given me that purpose.

The 'hole' was further filled when I became involved with Alice's story on *Emmerdale*. When I was searching for a publisher for this book I sought every avenue to bring this about. I offered a condensed version of my story to Cancer Research UK who were only too happy to accept and put it on their website under the title, *'Battles with Lymphoma'*. Eventually after many attempts I became discouraged. Some publishers would never reply, some would be highly critical, several would say they liked it but 'there was no room on their lists for another cancer story'. I felt dismayed and disgusted at the attitude of commercial publishers who were obviously only concerned about making money.

The search for a publisher made me feel stressed by early 2005 and my health seemed to suffer. Sarah told me to forget it. I came to the conclusion that it would never go into print.

One day in August I was talking to Sarah and we discussed how I finally felt fully recovered from the stem cell transplant. I was pleased to be well but life was not exciting any more. One week later Sarah shouted to me in an excited voice to check my e-mails. There was a message from a researcher at Granada Media who was researching for Emmerdale. She had seen my story on the Cancer Research UK website and informed me that the producers were planning a Non-Hodgkin's story in *Emmerdale*. Would I be willing to help them?

I danced around the room in excitement! This sounded very big. I might even become famous! I replied instantly and said that I would be very happy to help. A reply came back saying that they needed some extracts from the book to help the scriptwriters to write a realistic cancer story. It was to be about Alice, Sam Dingle's partner who would develop Non-Hodgkin's Lymphoma during pregnancy. I was also asked if I would be prepared to receive scripts from Granada Media and assess how realistic they were.

It was made clear that it would be on a voluntary basis but Granada Media would make a donation to a cancer charity at the end of the storyline. I was happy about this since I never aimed to make a penny from my illness. I decided that this donation should go to Dr Haynes' Lymphoma Trust Fund at Nottingham City Hospital which is one of the beneficiary charities of this book.

Between August and December I received scripts and in some cases they were very inaccurate. My consultant Dr Haynes was also involved on one occasion when the scriptwriters needed a specialist medical opinion.

The interest from *Emmerdale* revived my enthusiasm to seek a publisher for the book, anticipating much more interest now. However, I was to be disappointed again after contacting more publishers. By December Sarah and I became concerned that the book would not be in print when Alice's story really hit the screens. We wanted to maximise the sales to gain the highest possible level of donations for the cancer charities. I decided to ask Granada Media for permission to seek some publicity to help find a publisher. This was granted just before Christmas. However it actually came about through Sarah's own success.

During my illness Sarah continued her studying. I encouraged it to keep life as normal as possible. Between 2003 and 2005 she completed her A level law exams with an overall grade A achieving one of the Criminal Law modules at A2 with 100%. I thought that this was amazing and so apparently did her college who nominated her for an award. Sarah received this on 20 December 2005 at Broxtowe College, Nottingham. That evening Peter Jordan, a photographer working as a freelance for the *Nottingham Evening Post*, took a particular interest in Sarah's story. He took extra photographs of myself, Sarah and Dominic. We mentioned the book and *Emmerdale* and this was passed on to the *Nottingham Evening Post*. There was a telephone call from a reporter the next day and following this a photographer came to our home. The article duly appeared on page three on 30 December. That same day *Central News East* contacted me and the television cameras were in our home in the afternoon. Sarah and I were interviewed and the report was broadcast on 3 January 2006. We then had a short holiday and on arriving back the *Derbyshire Times* produced a further report on 12 January. This was followed by a huge two page article in the *Derby Evening Telegraph* on

20 January. A remarkable month was then complete with live interviews on *BBC Radio Nottingham* on 25 January when Ursula Marsden was linked up on air. This was followed by another interview on *BBC Radio Derby* on the Breakfast show the next day.

It seemed incredible that all of this had happened after the dark days of my illness. It seemed that something positive had already come from my illness.

However there are also negative aspects to the legacy from my illness. One of these is my intolerance of other human beings who abuse their bodies through excessive smoking, drinking and drugs. Lymphoma cancers are not caused by any of these although certain other cancers may be. I know that I should not judge other people on these grounds and people have free will to do what they wish but when you have experienced a cancer through no fault of your own, it is hard not to. I feel anger and resentment when I see people behaving in this way and I see their apparent immunity from harm, despite the way they live.

I also feel anger and resentment towards people who behave horribly to other people yet who never seem to suffer themselves. Many times Sarah and I get annoyed when someone behaves badly or has a repugnant, arrogant attitude. It is hard for us not to conclude that such a person has clearly never suffered any major problems or illnesses in their lives or they would not behave in such a way. This may or may not be true but it is the way we feel after everything which has happened in our lives. I also become very angry when I see the senseless killing by terrorists. These people do not understand how precious human life should be.

No-one is perfect in this world but every fellow cancer sufferer that I have met has appeared to be a 'decent' person. That is not to say that 'good' or 'nice' people always develop cancer nor to say that no people who behave badly develop the illness. Maybe it is that when someone develops cancer they change for the better and perhaps I have just never seen the bad side to them.

Sarah says she often assumes that other people do not have problems because they are looking cheerful. It is not that we have a chip on our shoulders about this but it can be hard to see people laughing when you may not feel like laughing, without creeping feelings of resentment; without feeling, why can't everything in our lives be as good as it seems to be for them? However many times you discover that the person behind the smile does indeed have their sorrows in life. Everyone has ups and downs in life and many families encounter cancer in some way. It is inevitable though that sometimes it just felt as though our family was the only one to be experiencing such unhappiness.

Thankfully, these feelings have faded after all of the exciting events which have happened.

As you might imagine, our faith in God has been tested generally. In fact, when I was in the Derbyshire Royal Infirmary in November and December 2003, I was visited by the Hospital Chaplain. He offered sympathy and prayers and in our discussions I described to him all of the events which had happened to Sarah and I over the years since 1991. His comment was, 'I'm surprised you have any faith left'.

However, we both believe that there was a positive force helping Sarah and myself to get through all these experiences. There was a great deal of prayer taking place at our local Baptist church and at Birkdale School. We are very grateful for these prayers and feel that they made a positive contribution to my recovery.

It has also been hurtful to hear stories of people expressing opinions about cancer which were misguided at best, and downright insulting at times. When I chatted to fellow cancer sufferers in clinics and wards I heard many such tales. The most disturbing one was from a lady who was suffering from leukaemia whom I met at Derby. She told me that her neighbour was selling up her house to move away from her because she believed that you could catch cancer like a cold. Words could not describe the anger I felt about this.

Sarah and I ourselves also encountered a form of discrimination. Unfortunately ignorance can cause this to happen with some people. We forgave them for this.

This brings me to the final aspect of the illness: the effect on the career or spouse and family as a whole. My son, Dominic, was very young through my illness and, thankfully, does not seem to have been affected by it all. When you are only six or seven years old your priorities are very different.

Sarah coped remarkably well each time I experienced the illness and the treatments which went with it. When I was diagnosed for the third time she believed that she just wouldn't be able to cope but she did. Carers or spouses are often forgotten and it is the cancer sufferer who receives all of the sympathy. Sarah has also volunteered to be a listener for partners with the Lymphoma Association.

I will never know the full truth of the emotional and physical pressure that Sarah was under during my treatments. There were the many hospital visits which were so very important to me in keeping up my morale. There was also the extra physical pressure of having to do more for me and around the house when I became weak. I have no doubt also that Sarah experienced many emotions and worries which she would not display to me because it might not help me get through.

There were also the emotions and feelings of my parents and brothers. During my illness I never really gave much thought to these compared to Sarah's and Dominic's feelings.

After my stem cell transplant I was offered rehabilitation group sessions by Nottingham City Hospital to discuss the treatments I had been through and their emotional effects. Both Sarah and I feel that such sessions should be available to carers and spouses as well and that is something that we should perhaps push for.

In conclusion, having cancer three times has been life-changing. Despite the negative feelings described earlier I feel that the whole experience has changed my life for the better and has made me a better person, although at the time it was actually happening I may not have appreciated this. I wanted my life to change for the better when I was too busy to have the time to do the things I really wanted to. I did not want that change to come about in the way it has but I am glad that it did.

Undoubtedly, it has left a scar, but it is essential to be positive and attempt to move on in your life each time. I live each day as it comes and try not to worry about the future. Some might say I have been unlucky to have cancer three times but I do not go through my life dwelling on this. There are people worse off than me in the world. Cancer is not necessarily a death sentence. In my case I regard it as a nuisance which I had to put up with just as Sarah has had to cope with her chronic fatigue and many other people have to cope with long-term conditions.

I have always maintained a positive attitude that the cancer can be beaten. It is not an easy road but with modern treatments and a will to come through, it can be overcome. I have learned the importance of never being afraid of the illness and of always believing, even when the going gets tough, that you will get better in the end.

I hope that this account of my experiences will be a help, and maybe even an inspiration, to others.